B7

£6·75

# Essentials of
# Child Psychiatry

D0533551

1 126449 00

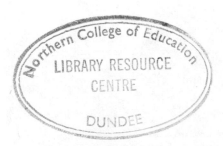

G

The b
Any t

90.

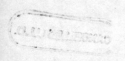

# Essentials of
# Child Psychiatry

## H. M. CONNELL

Senior Lecturer in
Child Psychiatry,
University of Queensland

FOREWORD BY
## J. G. P. RYAN

Professor of
Community Practice,
University of Queensland

BLACKWELL
SCIENTIFIC PUBLICATIONS
OXFORD LONDON EDINBURGH
MELBOURNE

© 1979 by Blackwell Scientific Publications
Osney Mead, Oxford, OX2 OEL
8 John Street, London, WC1N 2ES
9 Forest Road, Edinburgh, EH1 2QH
P.O. Box 9, North Balwyn, Victoria, Australia

First published 1979

**British Library Cataloguing in Publication Data**

Connell, H.M.
    Essentials of child psychiatry.
    1. Child psychiatry
    I. Title
    618.9'28'9    RJ499

    ISBN 0-632-00136-4

Distributed in U.S.A. by
Blackwell Mosby Book Distributors
11830 Westline Industrial Drive
St Louis, Missouri 63141,
in Canada by
Blackwell Mosby Book Distributors
86 Northline Road, Toronto
Ontario, M4B 3E5,
and in Australia by
Blackwell Scientific Book Distributors
214 Berkeley Street, Carlton
Victoria 3053

Typeset by Enset Ltd.
Midsomer Norton, Bath and
Printed and bound in Great Britain by
Billing & Sons Ltd, Guildford and Worcester.

# Contents

# Foreword

When I was asked to write a short foreword to what I consider to be a unique book in its field, I hoped that I was being asked as a general practitioner of 25 years standing, not as an academic of more limited experience. It has been my pleasure to assist Dr Connell in teaching during the last two years and to hear her lecturing to general practitioners on many occasions. It is always apparent that she is very conscious of the role of the general practitioner in the management of behavioural and minor psychiatric disorders in children, and appreciates the fact that the general practitioner, is as a result of his intimate knowledge of the family, in a favourable and privileged position to undertake this work. Indeed, it is probably true to say that if the doctor of first contact does not recognize psychopathology arising as a result of environmental and family stress it will probably go unrecognized, mis-diagnosed or untreated. Those of us interested in the discipline of general practice pay lip service to the concept of "whole person" medicine, and many of us practise this reasonably well, but I sometimes wonder whether in dealing with children we often tend to be too simplistic in our approach, and neglect the possible psychological factors that are either modifying the presentation of the illness or which in fact may be the underlying cause.

We perhaps have a tendency to look on our paediatric patients as rather uncomplicated and as a result of our traditional training often have an almost morbid fear of missing organic disease. As a result, psychological illness in children is almost invariably diagnosed by a long process of exclusion. It is unfortunate that the home visit is becoming increasingly less common in general practice. The family doctor can learn so much about a family in this setting and often it is easier to recognize that a 'sick' child is being presented as a call for help from a disturbed family.

Dr Connell's text is designed primarily for undergraduate medical students and is eminently readable; the illustrative case histories bring it to life. It is mercifully free of jargon, a very strong reason why it should appeal not only to readers from the medical and nursing professions but also to those in a wide variety of paramedical disciplines, such as social workers and medical psychologists as well as school teachers, child care workers and others involved in work with children. Intelligent parents, too, may find lucid explanations of many of the problems encountered in the very demanding task of raising children in the complex and threatening environment in which we are living. Most importantly, it has at last provided medical students with an excellent textbook to fill a gap in their training which has existed far too long.

As far as my general practitioner colleagues are concerned, this book should almost be obligatory reading. For those of them who are competent in this field, largely as a result of long experience, a human approach, and an almost intuitive ability to sense the complex disturbance that may lie behind the presentation of a childhood illness, the book will help them to integrate and reinforce their knowledge.

For those of them whose performance perhaps falls short of the ideal, as a result of pressure of work or inadequate training in this area of paediatrics in the first place, it is to be hoped that after reading this book they will see each and every paediatric problem in their practices through different eyes.

It is futile to believe that there will ever be enough child psychiatrists to cope with all the childhood behaviour problems in the community, and there would appear to be no reason why the great majority of them cannot be dealt with at the primary care level. As a profession we should ensure that the public is not disappointed in their expectations.

In recent years general practitioners especially in the city have had to relinquish some of their traditional skills, for example major surgery and anaesthesia. These have to be replaced by new skills which will eventually be recognized as just as rewarding and satisfying. I believe that Dr Connell's book offers the practitioner a very sound basic training in one of those new fields. May it have the success that it deserves.

# Preface

The psychological disorders of childhood are assuming importance in medical practice and attracting community concern generally. The need to include their study in medical courses is obvious. This book, based on lectures given to medical students and to family doctors, attempts to give an overview of such disorders, their aetiology, management and prevention. Although it has therefore a medical bias, it is hoped that it may be of assistance to other professionals involved with the welfare of children. It could also be used as an introduction to child psychiatry by candidates preparing for higher qualifications in psychiatry, and because of this, a reasonably wide bibliography is given for each chapter and in an appendix. However, emphasis is placed on the practical management of the child in his family, especially by the general practitioner, and most references cited are readily available. Realising that psychiatry may lend itself to jargon, terminology has, I hope, been kept as clear and simple as possible.

It is impossible to deal adequately with the complexity and richness of family life and its problems without clinical examples. Indeed, as Alice in Wonderland said, 'What is the use of a book without pictures and illustrations ?' I have, therefore, included illustrative case histories at the end of each chapter. In publications such as this, one is continually faced with the dilemma of describing clinical situations accurately, while respecting the confidentiality of the doctor–patient relationship. Every effort has therefore been made to disguise the identities of the patients, while keeping sufficient information to make the case studies worthwhile. I hope that no one will be able to recognize himself or others, and if by any chance some do, that they will forgive me, realizing that through teaching others they are helping with the treatment of families whose problems are close to their own.

Since a preface traditionally gives an opportunity to express gratitude, I would like to thank the countless children—and their parents—who have taught me, Mr P.G.Jones, whose surgical skill has pruned away non-essentials and Mrs T.Wright and Mrs E.Donovan, who typed the manuscript and whose patience lasted to the bitter end.

# Chapter 1

# The Evolution of Child Psychiatry and its Status Today
# Children in Trouble and How They Can be Helped
# Preventive Measures

'Do you know who made you?' 'Nobody as I knows of' said the child, with a short laugh . . . 'I 'spect I grow'd.'

Harriet Beecher Stowe (1812–1896)
*Uncle Tom's Cabin*

Child psychiatry, a comparative newcomer among medical specialties, has its roots in several disciplines, the chief being *paediatrics*, *adult psychiatry*, *psychology* and *education*. It developed as the result of:
● The recognition that the child's psychological development merited attention, as well as his physical.
● The hope that early intervention might alleviate some of the problems of adult mental disorder.

## THE BACKGROUND

The education and training of children in antiquity related chiefly to those of noble birth destined to fill important roles in adult life. Little attention was paid to childhood as a period when lifelong patterns of behaviour were laid down. Infants were of little concern as their hold on life was tenuous. When they could live without constant attention of mother or nurse, children were regarded as miniature adults and were expected to assume responsibility in the adult world, c.f. early paintings which depict children with adult proportions (Ariés 1960). Children were regarded as chattels and child marriages arranged to suit the convenience of families were not uncommon.

1

With the coming of the industrial revolution, children were exploited as a cheap source of labour. The Earl of Shaftsbury's crusade for improved working hours resulted in an 'enlightened' law which was passed over savage opposition in 1833. Children between nine and thirteen were not allowed to work more than a 48 hour week, those between thirteen and eighteen not more than 68 hours. Unfortunately, this rule did not apply to children in the mines, many of whom were crippled by lack of sunlight and desperately hard work. In England physical conditions were appalling for large numbers of children living in towns. In the eighteenth century it was estimated that a child born in London had only a fifty percent chance of survival beyond his fifth birthday, and the death rate was even higher in the large industrial towns of the north. Aspin (1969) reports that in Liverpool, England, in 1840, sixty-two percent of the population died before the age of five years. When the struggle for physical survival was so great, it is not surprising that the child's psychological development received scant attention.

Social conditions for children in the first settlement at Sydney Cove in 1788 were no better although there is some evidence that the 'bountious sunshine' of the Antipodes compensated to a degree (rickets was unknown), but food was limited and the diet unsuitable. A disproportionate number of the child population were born to unmarried convict women and the quality of care they received was questionable. Problem families appear to have been recognised by the administration and attempts made to help their children. In 1789 a 4-year-old girl was removed from the care of her mother (described as an abandoned woman), in order to save her from 'inevitable ruin' and sent to Norfolk Island to be taught reading, writing and husbandry (Gandevia & Gandevia 1975).


## THE DISCOVERY OF CHILDHOOD

During the nineteenth century there was a growing interest in childhood and recognition of its importance as a period of preparation for adult life. Scientists became concerned with individual records, for example, Charles Darwin described the day to day development of his own child. In the 1880's Stanley Hall studied thousands of parent questionnaires relating the behaviour of their offspring. On investigations such as these the foundations of developmental psychology were laid.

# RECOGNITION OF
# PSYCHOLOGICAL DISTURBANCE IN CHILDHOOD

Later, sporadic observations were made on deviant childhood behaviour. The difference between *mental subnormality* and *mental illness* in children was recognised. In France, Seguin experimented with methods of educating mentally deficient children and showed that their performance could be improved. In England Henry Maudsley (1867) described the development of insanity in early life. The first description of an autistic child was made by Haslam in 1799 (Walk 1964). A boy of ten years was studied at the Bethlem Hospital in London. He suffered a change in character at two, became the unrelenting foe of all glass, china and crockery, incapable of forming relationships and inaccessible to any display of kindness.

Management of severely disturbed children was often harsh since they were held morally responsible for their behaviour. In 1850, Crichton-Browne recommended a humane approach; a wholesome diet, cod liver oil and general cleanliness were to replace the lash and solitary confinement. Controversy about the nature of psychiatric disturbance in childhood was considerable. Kraft-Ebing and Heller postulated an organic basis, i.e. physical (brain) deterioration. Later, when higher education for women raised fears that female intellects might be over-taxed with knowledge, scholastic overstrain gained support as a cause of mental breakdown.

In 1911 Bleuler clarified the concept of schizophrenia; although his observations related chiefly to adult life, he suggested that this disorder could develop in childhood as early as the age of seven.

## THE TWENTIETH CENTURY

Kanner (1972) describes the evolution of ideas relating to the mental health of children and services designed to promote it, in this century, as follows:

### The first decade

During this period people began to think about children and their individual differences.

● *Compulsory school attendance* showed that some pupils were unable to profit by standard teaching. In Paris Binet, later assisted by Simon, devised a series of tests (subsequently known as intelligence tests) which differentiated such children from their peers. This allowed individual rates of maturation to be catered for in the educational system.

● Freud's studies of disturbed adults pointed to early childhood experiences as the root of their difficulties. With this came the realisation that such experiences should be studied first hand. This *dynamic approach*, i.e. explaining the origins of present disturbance in the past life of the individual, stressed the importance of a detailed biography as a means of understanding deviant behaviour.

● *The establishment of juvenile courts*, one was started in South Australia in 1895, removed children from the formality and punitive atmosphere of the adult judicature and created a need for workers both to help them and to learn why they had transgressed.

● Advances in bacteriology at that time had made *preventive measures* possible as regards physical disease. Could mental ill health be similarly prevented? If such was the case, then attention to childhood experiences became even more important. It was with the hope that adult psychiatric disturbance could be reduced or prevented by treating children showing deviant behaviour that child psychiatric services were first developed.

### The second decade

This was marked by serious efforts to understand childhood problems and, through community measures, to help those showing deviant behaviour:

● If a judge found a child guilty, *a period of probation* could be arranged when the child received guidance rather than punishment.

● *Foster home placement* became possible if a child's natural home was considered detrimental to his well-being.

● *Special classes* were developed to cater for those unable to profit by teaching in the general classroom.

### The third decade

Activity was now directed toward doing things for children in the family and school. Efforts were made to help children with 'everyday' problems with a view to preventing serious disturbance later on.

● *Child Guidance clinics* were established, starting with the Boston Habit Clinic in 1921.

● Because of the complex nature of many childhood problems *a multidisciplinary approach* by psychiatrist, social worker and psychologist evolved.

● Wickman drew attention to the need to involve teachers in the recognition of emotional and social problems in their pupils. *Parent–teacher organisations* developed and worked toward material improvements in the school environment.

### The fourth decade

Methods of working *with* problem children were now developed.

● Attention was paid to understanding *the individual child*, the meaning he attached to life events and why certain symptoms developed. Attempts were made to discover the conflicts underlying his disturbance and to help him resolve them. Because of the difficulties in communicating with young children verbally, Anna Freud and Melanie Klein pioneered the use of play as a means of communication and emotional release.

● The introduction of psychiatric departments into childrens' hospitals necessitated the liaison between several disciplines. A *whole child approach* became possible, physical and psychological care could be given simultaneously.

● In 1935 the first child psychiatric text was published by Leo Kanner; the revised edition of this still remains a reference today.

## FAMILIES IN TROUBLE

### The child

Disturbed children don't come asking for help themselves. They are generally brought by parents, or referred by teachers, social agencies or even the police. Understandably this may make for reluctance on the child's part and this must be allowed for. A child is often unaware of what is troubling him and even if he were, would be unlikely to discuss his problems freely with a stranger. One is therefore, dependent on how adults perceive a behavioural disturbance, at least in the initial stages of contact.

Broadly, psychopathology in childhood falls into three areas:
● Development/learning difficulties—often with an 'organic' basis (*neurophysiological disorder*).
● Emotional/behavioural problems—generally these appear to be *reactive* to environmental stresses of various sorts.
● *Psychophysiological disorders*—the child responds to stress with somatic symptoms.

Aetiological factors therefore relate to adverse psychological factors (both emotional and sociocultural), physical disorders (especially with central nervous system involvement) and less certainly, genetic predisposition. However, childhood disturbance is very commonly *multifactorial*, i.e. produced by the interaction of several factors. Even when the disturbance lies primarily in the child, his family's attitudes and management will influence considerably the clinical picture. It follows, that if childhood disturbance is reactive in nature or has a large reactive component, it should be potentially reversible and a positive and confident approach to its management is justified.

*The symptom*

Children don't complain of their feelings, e.g. of being depressed or anxious, but tend to show their emotions through behaviour, 'acting out' their feelings. In physical illness one symptom, may have many causes, so may one type or behaviour in a child. For example, stealing may be associated with an attempt to get 'kicks' from outwitting shopkeepers, with parental models who steal, with a need to buy popularity by giving presents, with a genuine lack of material possessions, or may be an unconscious attempt to compensate for rejection on the part of parents. Often parents expect immediate relief of symptoms without regard for the underlying causes. They may need help to appreciate that unless attention is paid to the basic disturbance, substitution of one type of deviant behaviour by another, *symptom substitution*, may occur.
Symptoms commonly described by parents are:
● *Slowness*—delay in passing developmental milestones, later difficulty in keeping up at school.
● *Naughtiness*—attention-getting, negativism, restlessness, aggression.
● *Sickness*—when psychological disturbance is expressed through somatic symptoms especially headache and abdominal pain.
● *Nervousness*—shyness, signs of anxiety, sleep disturbance.

## The parents

Parents may feel guilty about the need to seek help—'there are no disturbed children, only disturbed parents'—dies hard. Most try to be good parents but are hampered by their own personalities and up-bringing and are therefore unduly sensitive to criticism. Many hope for an immediate solution to longstanding difficulties, some that they will be relieved of the responsibility of managing the child's misbehaviour or even that the child be removed from their care. Others expect to have their punitive attitudes reinforced. Overall families who bring children for help fall into three groups:

1   Those where the *disturbance is primarily in the child*, e.g. a child with brain damage who presents with learning problems.

2   Those where there is little wrong with the child but parents run into difficulties because of their own inadequacies or neurotic difficulties. Thus the child is the *presenting symptom of a disturbed family*.

3   Very commonly, a *combination of 1 and 2*, e.g. an overactive aggressive child whose shy, easily depressed mother reacts to boisterous behaviour with timidity and inconsistency making him insecure, thus increasing his restlessness and agression.

Since there are varying degrees of child and parental disturbance in any family and the nuisance value of a symptom often determines the attention it receives (noisiness and aggression are more difficult to live with than shyness and withdrawal), the newcomer to child psychiatry must learn to evaluate the extent of the child's disturbance objectively and not be unduly influenced by parents.

## The role of the family doctor

Obviously this depends upon individual orientation but can be very important. The family doctor often has an intimate knowledge of the child's background which clinic staff would find hard to obtain and parents prefer to take him into their confidence rather than discuss their difficulties with strangers. We have already seen that

*Behaviour disorder = child + family*

A family doctor, interested in human behaviour and relationships has therefore much to offer the disturbed family. His strength lies in sup-portive care, in giving:

● *Explanation.* Helping parents develop insight into why their child behaves as he does.
● *Advice.* Practical easily understood suggestions about management.
● *Reassurance.* Restoring parents confidence in their ability to cope.
Above all he is someone who is known and can be consulted in a crisis. This may be of more value than sophisticated treatment, in many cases.

No one leaves their childhood behind entirely. Contact with disturbed families inevitably reawakens long forgotten conflicts associated with one's own childhood. It is important to remember that this child-of-years-gone-by may still affect clinical judgement and to be on the alert for this when working with children (see p. 54, developing insight).

## PEOPLE WHO WORK WITH DISTURBED CHILDREN: A TEAM APPROACH

A multidisciplinary team comprising psychiatrist, psychologist, social worker, play therapist and often a remedial teacher is usual in the management of disturbed children within a clinic setting. Other professionals such as speech therapists and physiotherapists may be involved as well. When children are treated in an in-patient unit, nursing staff join the team. The need for a team reflects the multi-determined nature of childhood disorder and a 'whole child' approach. Needless to say adequate communication between all members is essential. Although roles are not rigidly defined, the psychiatrist is generally concerned with the management of the case and the mental and physical examination of the child, the psychologist with assessment of the child's cognitive ability and personality traits, and the social worker with the background from which the child comes. All three may be involved in psychotherapy with the child or his parents (see p. 11). The play therapist and teacher direct their efforts primarily toward the child.

## THE PRESENT STATUS OF PSYCHIATRIC SERVICES FOR CHILDREN

In the past three decades child psychiatry has become a well established entity with clinical, teaching and research commitments. In the clinical field, work is centred on child psychiatric clinics and psychiatric departments of childrens' hospitals. Centres catering for disturbed adolescents are a newer and important development. Liaison with paediatricians, general practitioners, childrens' courts, and with welfare and education departments are an essential part of a clinic's work.

Hopes that early treatment of deviant behaviour in child psychiatric clinics would reduce the prevalence of adult mental disorder have not been realised (Rutter 1972). Nevertheless much disturbed behaviour in childhood appears to be reactive to environmental events and merits early and energetic attention. Escalation of problems upon a primary disturbance in child or family (the vicious spiral) is common and by the time help is sought, the situation is compounded and treatment may be made more difficult. Conventional methods of management in clinics are often time consuming, and this, together with shortages of trained staff, has resulted in long waiting lists and criticism of services. There is evidence that disturbed families in poor socio-economic circumstances do not visit clinics as much as they need, whereas middle-class families receive more than their share of a clinic's time (Eisenberg 1969). With these factors in mind, some child psychiatrists are shifting their orientation from the individual child in a clinic setting to community oriented programmes in order to ensure early intervention and a reduction of the demands made on clinics. This is not to deny the necessity of individual treatment for the seriously disturbed; the aim is to utilise psychiatric staff as effectively as possible.

Community programmes involve the education of all who work with children about the needs of the growing personality and the likely consequences of their not being met. Faced with major social problems involving young people, such as delinquency, violence and broken families, some workers turn to child psychiatry hoping for an answer as to why these occur. Unfortunately, the child psychiatrist is in no stronger a position than anyone else to suggest a solution. Nevertheless, research into early personality development and the origins of deviant behaviour are important areas for child psychiatry.

## THE PSYCHIATRIC TREATMENT
## OF CHILDREN

Ways and means of helping the disturbed child and his family are described as a preliminary to studying clinical syndromes. However it is suggested that reference be made to this section while other chapters are being read.

## General principles

● *Careful history-taking* is an essential to starting treatment. The child
and his environment must be considered together. Other family members
may need help, e.g. it is useless giving tranquillisers to a child because
his neurotically depressed mother cannot cope with normal childhood
behaviour.

● From knowledge derived from the history, *a plan can be formulated*
and a decision made as to what is remediable and how it can be changed.
Where unalterable factors exist, the child must be helped to cope with
them.

● Treatment should *interfere as little as possible with normal activities.*
If it necessitates repeated absences from school, the consequent educational handicap could aggravate the primary disturbance.

## The first interview can be therapeutic

If parents can ventilate their anxieties in the presence of an adviser who
does not regard them as foolish nor condemn them for failure, help can
be given at the start of contact with the family. Parents can be reassured
perhaps, that the child's behaviour is not as abnormal as they thought,
and that other parents have similar problems. As they talk through their
difficulties they may develop insight into what has gone wrong and why.
In his first encounter with a member of the clinic staff, a child may be
helped to realise that he is not 'queer' or 'bad', and that he has an ally
in his therapist, who is genuinely concerned in seeing family problems
objectively and helping him with personal difficulties. He may speak
freely to an adult as never before when he learns the confidential nature
of the professional relationship.

## Reduction of environmental stress

Factors which appear to produce or aggravate disturbed behaviour may
relate to:

● *School.* Discussion with the child's teacher will often clarify *classroom
problems.* Remedial help or transfer to a more appropriate class or school
may be necessary.

● *Home.* Efforts to improve *parental attitudes* toward the child and practical advice regarding management can be very important. Occasionally parents may require psychiatric referral. If parent figures are absent substitute care may have to be provided.

● *Social environment.* Group activities such as youth clubs, Scouts and Guides and holiday camps can be invaluable for socially inhibited children as well as those whose families offer little support and opportunities for creative activities.

## Psychotherapy

This form of treatment is based upon the relationship between a professionally trained person (the therapist) and the patient. There are several types of psychotherapy reflecting different ideologies, but the common basis is that *through interpersonal communication* (both verbal and non-verbal) in an interview situation, *the patient is helped to modify his attitudes and behaviour.*

The benefits of psychotherapy for a child result from:

● An opportunity to ventilate aggressive feelings and the anxiety which accompanies them in an understanding atmosphere where retaliation is not a constant threat.

● The therapist's encouragement of mature behaviour in lieu of maladaptive, infantile patterns which interfere with personality growth.

Experimental evidence for the value of psychotherapy is not easy to obtain, but there is no doubt that children benefit from contact with an understanding person with whom they can identify, who teaches that adults can be trusted and who encourages responsible attitudes and behaviour.

Some children, especially if severely disturbed, are best seen individually, others may find a one-to-one relationship with an adult too threatening and are more comfortable in a group of between 5–10 others. This has the advantages of economy as well as helping children with difficulties in social relationships. Group therapy with parents may be arranged simultaneously. Play is the natural way for a child to express his feelings and, especially with younger children, may be utilized in therapy sessions. Observation of play and creative activities (drawing, painting, modelling) gives the therapist insight and the same medium may be used as a means of communicating with the child.

Psychotherapy sessions last $1-1\frac{1}{2}$ hours and are generally held at weekly intervals. The therapist is usually a graduate of one of the behavioural sciences (psychology, social work, occupational therapy) but has additional psychotherapeutic training.

## Family therapy

Recognition of the family's part in the genesis and perpetuation of childhood behaviour disorder is long standing, however, the logical approach i.e. treating the child and his family together as a unit, is a comparatively recent development. Family therapy involves one or more members of the child's family being present during his sessions with the therapist. This allows the therapist to assess family functioning as a whole, to improve communication between family members and to help them develop insight as to why certain patterns of behaviour have emerged. If they can see these behaviours as maladaptive they may learn to cope better in the future. Although the underlying theoretical orientation may be psychoanalytic or behavioural or both and the therapists interpretations differ, the principle of interaction between family members in the presence of a neutral therapist is utilized whatever the orientation.

The indications for family therapy are (Graham 1976):
● Where the child's disturbance is clearly a manifestation of family disturbance.
● Where there is no improvement with individual therapy.
● Where treatment of one member produces stress or symptoms in other members.

Family therapy is generally considered to be contraindicated:
● When the family is in the process of breaking up.
● When the child's difficulties lie within himself (intrapsychic pathology).
● Where the child is reacting to stress outside the family e.g. to learning problems at school.

Although some regard severe and pervasive hostility between members a contraindication, this is not always so. Where conflict exists between the child and his parents, providing the therapist can take the strain, family therapy can be most helpful especially as the older child tends to see the therapist as siding with his parents if they are seen alone.

## Behaviour therapy

This approach, based upon experimentally established principles of learning has an accepted place in the management of childhood disturbance. The treatment of bedwetting by a method of conditioning is described in Chapter 9 Desensitization by exposing the child to a hierarchy of feared situations is also used, for example gradually bringing a child into closer and closer contact with some animal he fears. School refusal (see Chapter 7) can be treated this way, although a rapid return to the classroom can also be effective. Parents have modified their children's behaviour by positive and negative reinforcement (reward and punishment) since pre-history but the value of shaping behaviour using a scientifically planned programme has only recently gained recognition. Some speech disorders, social withdrawal in austistic children and attention-seeking behaviour can all be treated in this way. When using this method (operant conditioning) the emphasis is on positive reinforcement and social rewards (praise and encouragement) rather than negative reinforcement and material rewards. Generally psychologists undertake behaviour therapy but parents can be trained to be their children's therapists.

## Chemotherapy

Drugs play a small but useful part in the management of disturbed children: psychotherapy, chemotherapy and environmental manipulation must always go hand in hand. It is unfortunate that the English language does not distinguish between a drug of addiction and a drug with medical value. Many parents, quite rightly, question the wisdom of suggesting to a youngster that drugs can help with emotional difficulties, and ask about the chances of habituation. The answer must be that there is no clear evidence that drug dependent adults have been treated excessively with drugs in childhood, and that judicious short-term use of drugs in children may prevent the development of disorders which could predispose to drug abuse later. The principles of drug therapy and tables of dosage are listed in Appendix A. Most psychoactive drugs are highly toxic if taken in greater amounts than those prescribed. The potential danger for toddler siblings and the possibility of suicidal behaviour in the older child must be borne in mind.

## Help from other disciplines

Speech therapists and physiotherapists have a part to play in some disorders and in the management of particular symptoms. Occupational therapy has much to offer, giving the disturbed child a chance to work through his difficulties as he becomes involved in creative activity. Remedial teaching is often necessary and liaison with education authorities may be an essential part of treatment.

## *Social worker involvement with families* (casework)

The team approach to the management of disturbed children has already been described. Despite what has been said about family therapy, in some instances there are advantages in the child being the concern of one member, and his family of another. The child feels that his therapist sees his point of view and this contributes substantially to the development of satisfactory rapport. The same considerations apply to the child's family, who may have difficulties in their own right. In such circumstances a social worker can give assistance in discussing these and help in practical ways, for example as regards housing or monetary allowances as well as interpreting treatment offered to the child at the clinic.

## *In-patient treatment*

So far, treatment described has been based on an out-patient basis. This has much to commend it. Parents can be seen when they bring the child and family members can work through their difficulties together. Reasons for admission to a residential unit, which is generally associated with a hospital, are:

● For *diagnostic work-up*. This is particularly useful under Australian conditions where home may be a long way from hospital. The effects of treatment can be observed at the same time.

● Where severe disturbance makes *management at home impossible* e.g. aggressive behaviour disorders, depression with hints of suicide, psychotic disturbance.

● If the child's physical state requires *skilled nursing care* as in anorexia nervosa (see Chapter 12).

● Where adverse environmental circumstances are such that it is felt no improvement can be expected if the child remains *in situ*.

● Where there is gross overprotection by parents or encouragement of invalidism after illness or injury.

● Where the treatment of school refusal has failed and the child can be reintroduced to school from the unit rather than from home.

If admission is necessary every effort must be made to maintain family ties during the child's stay. There is much to be said for admitting the mother, with the child if he is of pre-school age. Observation of mother–child interaction may make diagnosis easier and it gives an opportunity to demonstrate improved methods of management to the mother.

The milieu of the unit should encourage social interaction and responsible behaviour. Children must be helped to understand that the staff have great sympathy for their difficulties, are there to help them cope, and not to punish. Children should be accepted warmly but it must be made clear that for the safety of themselves and others, limits are necessary. Opportunities must be given for work and play as at home. Daily attendance at school (sometimes one is run in conjunction with the unit) and recreational activity after school hours is essential. Good communication between members of the staff is most necessary and a short 'team meeting' after the children have left for school is an important part of the day's activities.

While he is away from home, work with his family is essential to prevent the child's return to the same difficulties he experienced before. Generally this is undertaken by a social worker attached to the unit.

### Day patient treatment

Where geography permits this may be an alternative to admission in some cases. It may also be desirable following discharge from hospital where a gradual integration into family life is needed.

## WAYS OF REDUCING PSYCHIATRIC DISTURBANCE IN CHILDREN

### Traditional concepts in preventive work

Three levels are generally recognised at which intervention may reduce the prevalence of mental ill-health:

● *Primary prevention.* This is involved with amelioration of harmful influences likely to produce mental ill health, for example, the provision of good obstetric care or helping families in poor social circumstances.

● *Secondary prevention* is aimed at reducing the prevalence of disease by early detection and prompt treatment. An example of this would be

the screening of school children for learning difficulties and instituting remedial work before negative attitudes to school develop.
● *Tertiary prevention.* This attempts to minimise the effects of residual disabilities and to take advantage of remaining assets after mental disorder has been recognised and treated; rehabilitation and follow-up services are important in this connection. The re-integration of the brain injured child into school and society is an example.

## Recognition of the child at risk

Preventing maladjustment from developing at all is obviously the ideal but would be very hard to accomplish. Although further research into aetiological factors is most necessary, recognition of children at risk of developing psychiatric disturbance is possible.

In the sections which follow we shall look at the possibilities for detecting vulnerable children and ways in which they can be helped. This is really a combination of primary and secondary prevention.

## Hereditary factors

Our present state of knowledge does not allow us to predict hereditary predisposition to psychiatric disorder in childhood, although we have some knowledge of genetic factors in adult mental illness. Certain types of mental subnormality are known to have a hereditary basis (see Chapter 11) and in these cases parents can be helped to understand facts and get them in perspective. Aside from this, many parents of disturbed children benefit greatly from discussing their fears, often irrational, regarding sinister genetic influences, and this is the time when the importance of environment and upbringing can be pointed out to them. The family doctor is often in an ideal position to do this.

## Antenatal care

Good obstetric care involves attention to physical and psychological aspects of pregnancy, and reduces the likelihood of abnormality or disturbance in the child. It includes:
● Prevention of diseases in the mother known to affect the foetus, e.g. rubella. Ensuring adequate nutrition during pregnancy.

● Early detection of abnormalities likely to affect delivery.
● Attention to the mother's emotional health and her preparation for parenthood.
● Education of both parents as to the psychological needs of the child.

## Preventive measures in infancy

Improved techniques in the care of neonates, especially if premature, have resulted in an increased survival rate, and in general lessened the incidence of severe handicaps. However, some survivors of perinatal difficulties may suffer from subtle defects which are not immediately obvious, and 'at risk' registers have been developed for follow-up of likely cases. These have proved a mixed blessing. They do contribute to early detection but tend to make parents anxious and, overprotective and to look for problems where none exist. Screening infants for signs of handicap e.g. cerebral palsy and for inborn errors of metabolism e.g. phenylketonuria are important in order to institute early treatment.

When parents are unable to care for their child, fostering or adoption, depending on circumstances, avoids the sequelae of early emotional deprivation (see Chapter 6). Since the number of young babies available for adoption has dropped in recent years, the opportunity to select adoptive parents is better than previously.

## Preventive measures in the pre-school years

Screening tests have been devised to detect children with handicaps likely to impair school performance (see Chapter 9). These must also be employed judiciously otherwise parents and teachers may anticipate difficulties too readily and fail to appreciate that many maturational lags improve with time. The establishment of pre-school centres in areas where socially disadvantaged families live, can result in improved physical health, adjustment and social skills of young children. Unfortunately children from the most necessitous families often attend sporadically or not at all. This is particularly true of Aboriginal families living in urban surroundings. Measures to attract such children are needed.

Parental maladjustment has a major impact upon the lives of offspring especially in the early years. Early detection of families with a high potential for child abuse can lead to effective prevention (Lynch *et al.* 1976). Depressive symptoms in a mother sometimes develop as the result of social isolation ('suburban neurosis') and can be particularly damaging. The establishment of play groups, run largely by voluntary effort has helped many. Children have space and companionship and mothers an opportunity for social interaction. A roster of mothers allows them some freedom to go shopping or whatever. In Australia the value of these groups for migrant families is considerable, especially as language classes for mothers can be run concurrently.

### Programmes for the school child

Early detection can prevent much of the secondary emotional disturbance associated with learning difficulties. Guidance officers from State education departments can screen children, institute remedial work, and advise on appropriate placement if a change of class or school is indicated. Remedial work should involve both academic and emotional aspects, attention being given to the lack of self-confidence generated by learning problems.

Teachers may need help in recognising the symptoms of emotional disturbance in childhood and how to approach interpersonal difficulties in the classroom.

In secondary schools, a school counsellor able to advise on vocational choice will help to prevent problems of getting into an unsuitable academic stream. Staff should be aware of the early signs of drug abuse and of serious psychiatric disturbance in adolescence and where help can be found. Social experience for the isolated youngster can be provided by the establishment of youth groups, fitness camps and other peer group activities. Sex education in schools must be tackled seriously if it is to improve the attitudes and adjustment of youngsters. Its potential to reduce the incidence of venereal disease in adolescence and teenage pregnancies cannot be ignored.

### Mitigating the effects of poverty

Physical and psychological problems beset the child from an impoverished background. Poor housing, inadequate nutrition, lack of social stimulation, family tensions, incompetence and disruption can all be tackled. Help at the pre-school level has already been described, but this has to be followed up if improved adjustment is to be maintained. However, the basic question is—how and when can cycles of deprivation be interrupted and one generation after another of socially incompetent families be prevented ? There is no simple answer. Improvement in material conditions only helps to some extent. Housing may be changed with little difficulty, but attitudes and a way of life, not so easily.

Social worker involvement with such families and assistance with all aspects of existence, budgeting, nutrition and contraceptive advice, as well as education about the basic needs of children, can be of value. Until research answers some of the questions relating to 'multi-problem' families this is certainly the best approach.

## *Summary*

The prevention of mental ill health in childhood is an investment for the future, and should be given the attention it merits. Much work remains to be done in improving community attitudes toward the needs of children and to ensure that help is sought before disorders become ingrained. The prevention, early detection and treatment of psychiatric disorder in children is not the exclusive province of child psychiatrists but involves family doctors, paediatricians, teachers and all whose work involves contact with children. It is hoped this book will increase their interest and awareness of the subject.

## CLINICAL EXAMPLE

The following is an account of a visit made by a mother and her eight year old son to a psychiatric outpatient department. It illustrates the interaction of factors which make child psychiatry the interesting subject it is.

Peter lives in a comfortable suburban home with his mother and grandmother. His mother sought an appointment because she felt she couldn't cope with him any more. She had already visited a Child Guidance Clinic, her family doctor on many occasions, and a private neurologist. The mother was a very neatly dressed woman of forty-six years. She brought a written list of complaints about her son.

### *This is what she told the doctor:*

MOTHER: I just can't manage him. He's hyperactive. He threw a spade at an old man, and hit an old lady in the stomach. He's spilled water on my new carpet and knocked over china things and broke them. He makes a mess when he eats, he won't tidy up. He won't do anything I ask him to. He's jealous of anything I care about and is rough with my little cat; it was sick so I took it to the vet and he said it had been hit on the head. I know Peter did it.

DOCTOR: Did you see him do it?

MOTHER: No but he's just so rough. He's stolen things from me too. Biscuits from the kitchen, money from my purse, to buy lollies. He's always asking me if I love him and if I'm going to hospital again.

DOCTOR: Have you been to hospital recently?

MOTHER: Yes, I've got chest trouble (bronchiectasis) and been in hospital several times. When I was pregnant with Peter I was in hospital for treatment on and off most of the time. They tried me in labour, but after a long time did a Caesar. I was thirty-eight you see when he was born. I married at thirty-six and it took two years to get pregnant.

DOCTOR: Did you have any drugs during the pregnancy?

MOTHER: No, only antibiotics and something to help me sleep. He was always a difficult baby. He wouldn't feed properly and was always screaming and windy. When he was a toddler he never seemed to settle and had bad screaming attacks when he wanted something and I wouldn't give it to him. He's always fidgety and gets worked up. He doesn't sleep well. Early this year he kept getting stomach pains and vomiting and missed school because of this. In the morning, he just used to bring up spit and looked pale. He's always been sickly and has been attending doctors since he was born. Then they sent him to remedial classes and he got better. When he was little— three years ago he had Perthes's Disease in his hip and he had crutches for seventeen months and he missed one year's schooling then. He's bad at writing and used to do letters the wrong way round—like 6 and 9 or p and q. He was at a private school, but was doing no good. He changed schools and has done better since then. He doesn't have any friends you see.

DOCTOR: Are there any boys around his home?

MOTHER: Yes, but they're a rough lot. I won't have them in the house— they break things—precious things—I've got a lovely home, my husband left me pretty well off.

DOCTOR: Father is dead then?

MOTHER: Yes, he died three years ago from cancer. They first told him he'd got it just after Peter was born, so he was sickly for most of

Peter's life, and we had to keep Peter quiet so he wouldn't make his father worse. I sent Peter away to friends when his father died. I was too upset you see. He keeps asking where his father has gone. I say to heaven. He asks when he'll come back but I can't bring myself to tell him it will be never.

DOCTOR: What do you say?

MOTHER: Oh I just change the subject and send him off to do something. My mother's very good. She's seventy-six and she spends a lot of time playing with Peter. He'll do things for her too. If I say one thing and she says another he does what she tells him.

DOCTOR: Do you argue over Peter?

MOTHER: Well, we try not to but there's only the three of us in the house and it's hard not to get on each others' nerves.

DOCTOR: Do you have bad nerves?

MOTHER: Yes, my family have too. After my husband died I got very upset. Not sleeping, couldn't eat, couldn't do anything in the home and usually I'm a very tidy, careful person. They gave me brown tablets.

DOCTOR: They?

MOTHER: The family doctor. My brother committed suicide just before my husband died. I felt I'd lost everything. All my family have nerves—my mother gets bad headaches when things go wrong. Peter needs a man in the house I know. He's always looking for someone. If a tradesman comes in he switches right off and goes to him. I couldn't ever marry again though, I worked in an office— really top secretarial job until I was thirty-six, then I married Peter's father who was forty-five. I was sorry to give up my career because I was so good at it. There's one thing keeps worrying me all the time though Doctor, I can't get it out of my mind. Peter's father had a brother who behaved like Peter when he was a boy. He's in an asylum now. Could it be the same thing? Is there something pressing in Peter's brain? I know Doctor Blank (the private neurologist) said there was nothing wrong but it keeps worrying me just the same. Should we have some more tests done?

DOCTOR: Has Peter had any fits?

MOTHER: No nothing like that, just always tense and clinging to me or getting angry and aggressive at me.

DOCTOR: Was he slow developmentally?

MOTHER: Well he was an only child and I didn't know about babies— never touched one before. I was the youngest of the family you see. But he stood up at one year, walked at eighteen months, said words at about one year, they thought he was OK at the Well Baby Clinic. His birth weight was $7\frac{1}{2}$ lbs.

### Examination of Peter

He appeared to be a normal eight year old, and related well, his verbal ability was good.

DOCTOR: Why did you come ?

PETER: Well Mum thinks I hurt her cat but I didn't, honest I didn't. She got mad at me for spilling the water too but I only knocked something over. I hate that old man—I know he tells Mum I've done things I haven't. He said I'd stole his mangoes and broke his tree but I didn't. They're all getting at me in the street. Granny's the only one who sticks up for me but she's boring, she's so old.

DOCTOR: Have you any friends ?

PETER: Well there's a few kids around but Mum says they're rough and we can't play in our yard. If I go out I have to tell Mum where I'll be playing and she comes to see If I'm there.

When asked about his father Peter said, 'He's dead', and then became angry and sullen and it was considered wiser not to press the subject further at that stage.

Throughout his session, Peter was tense and anxious, his palms were moist and at times he breathed heavily. It was noted that he was a clumsy, poorly co-ordinated child whose writing and attempts to copy geometric figures were very poor.

### The School report stated

Peter has been badly behind with school work, especially reading, but with remedial help this has improved. His attention span is very limited, he can't seem to concentrate. His behaviour with other children in the classroom isn't too bad, but in the playground he is aggressive and unpopular.

### Diagnosis

The reader may like to pick out some of the adverse factors which have affected this child for himself. It does not require a great deal of psychiatric expertise to do so. Here are some suggestions.

*1. Mother's attitude to Peter*
She is an excessively tidy, careful woman with a successful career before marriage. Peter was fretful and colicky and quite unlike the well behaved baby she would have wished for. He did not offer much compensation for the life she relinquished when she married. Moreover, soon after Peter's birth she was told of her husband's illness, and was in constant fear that Peter's crying would make his condition worse. She has little idea of the normal behaviour of children and obviously prizes her possessions above Peter's freedom. Peter lives in an atmosphere of divided authority; grandmother and mother approach him quite differently and argue over his management.

*2. Illness and death of father*
Peter has never known a father healthy enough to be a companion and may well have identified being a male with being sick. This would be exaggerated when he suffered from an orthopaedic condition requiring crutches, which placed him squarely in the invalid role. Subsequently when he found school adjustment difficult he became 'sick' and thus avoided going. His efforts to find male companions to replace the lost father have been continually frustrated by his mother who 'won't have rough boys in her beautiful home'. At the time of his father's death, Peter's idea of what had happened was vague and confused. He was sent away and when he returned found a withdrawn, depressed mother who has never at any time explained to him what death really means. Many children of his age show resentment at what they see as desertion by the deceased parent, some will blame the surviving parent for allowing the death to occur. Since Peter was conditioned early in life to keep quiet in order not to disturb his father he may well feel responsible for his father's death now, and guilty about it.

*3. Peter's attitudes*
There are many reasons for Peter feeling both anxious and angry. His mother's mixed feelings toward him, her absences in hospital (when he may fear she will disappear as his father did), her continual criticism, and his failure at school are a few. When he becomes angry he attacks others and invites rejection and retribution, in fact he has such a bad name now that he is expected to behave badly. All this serves to make him insecure, and in an effort to boost his morale he steals and tries to

draw attention to himself with silly, aggravating behaviour. This causes further rejection and the vicious circle continues.

## 4. Neurophysiological dysfunction

Peter's poor concentration, pattern of behaviour in infancy and clumsiness are common in children with a history suggestive of cerebral damage in early life. He was certainly a child 'at risk'. The mother was ill throughout pregnancy and labour was difficult. Moreover, she was thirty-eight at the time of his birth and there is known to be a higher incidence of complications in a first pregnancy as late as this. Detailed examination and psychological assessment later, confirmed minor neurological impairment.

## 5. Heredity

Although we do not know in many cases to what extent predisposition to psychiatric disturbance is inherited, on both sides of Peter's family there are individuals who seem to have been very disturbed. For example, one uncle committed suicide, another is permanently in a psychiatric hospital and the mother's rigid and perfectionistic personality traits are evident. She also gives a history of suffering from 'nerves'.

In the chapters that follow methods of assessing situations such as this, and of their management, especially within the setting of a family practice, will be described.

## References

ARIÈS P. (1960) *Centuries of Childhood*. Ringwood, Victoria: Penguin Books Australia Ltd. p. 125.

ASPIN C. (1969) *Lancashire: the First Industrial Society*. Preston, England, United Printing Services.

GANDEVIA B. & GANDEVIA S. (1975) Childhood mortality: its social background in the first settlement at Sydney Cove, 1788–1792. *Aust. Paed. J.* **11**, 9–19,

GRAHAM P. (1976) Management in child psychiatry: recent trends. *Brit. J. Psychiat.* **129**, 97–108.

EISENBERG L. (1969) Child psychiatry. The past quarter century. *Amer. J. Orthopsychiatry*, **39**, 389–401 (*Annual Progress*, Vol. 3, 1970*).

KANNER L. (1972) *Child Psychiatry* (4th ed). Springfield, Illinois, Charles C. Thomas. Chapter 1.

LYNCH M.A., ROBERTS J. & GORDON M. (1976) Child abuse: early warning in the maternity hospital. *Develop. Med. Child Neurol.* **18**, 759–766.

MAUDSLEY H. (1867) *Physiology and Pathology of the Mind*. New York, Appleton.

## General reading

RUTTER M. (1972) Relationships between child and adult psychiatric disorders. *Acta Psychiatrica Scandinavica*, **48**, 3–21 (*Annual Progress*, Vol. 6, 1973*).
PHAIRE T. (1545, 1955 reprint) *The Boke of Chyldren*. Edinburgh and London: E.S. Livingstone Ltd.
WALK A. (1964) The prehistory of child psychiatry. *Brit. J. Psychiatry*, **110**, 754,
* See Appendix B.

# Chapter 2

# Normal Psychological Development

'When I was one I had just begun
When I was two I was nearly new
When I was three I was hardly me
When I was four I was not much more
When I was five I was just alive
But now I am six I'm as clever as clever
I think I'll be six now for ever and ever.'

A. A. Milne
*Now We Are Six*

## THE 'NORMAL' CHILD

A knowledge of normal psychological development must be the basis for the appreciation of psychological disturbance in childhood. A child is regarded as 'normal' if his behaviour conforms to that of his peers. There are wide variations in childhood behaviour and it is often hard to decide where abnormality begins. Age, sex and intelligence must all be considered before labelling a child as 'deviant', as must the environment from which he comes. Compare the backgrounds of two children in contemporary Australia. One, whose father works in a professional sphere lives in a suburb where middle class families predominate. He has personal belongings, his own bed and bedroom, his health and diet are carefully watched, he is never left without an adult in charge of him, and is protected from some unsavory aspects of modern existence. The other, son of an itinerant labourer, lives in a large city in overcrowded, substandard housing. He shares a bedroom with several siblings and a bed with one or even more. Most of his clothes are handed down. He is frequently left alone, or to care for siblings barely younger than he is. He may know what it is to be hungry, and his knowledge of some of the physical aspects of human existence may be phenomenal. Understandably the behaviour shown by these children reflects the background to which each has adapted (middle class suburbia vs concrete jungle) and though very different, is not necessarily abnormal. Children must not be judged in isolation, and the observer must beware of relying on his own social mores and upbringing as a frame of reference.

# HUMAN DEVELOPMENT:
## BIOLOGICAL — PSYCHOLOGICAL — SOCIAL

It is convenient to consider a child's development as occurring simultaneously in these areas and there is generally close correlation between them. The mentally subnormal child is often physically and emotionally immature and lags behind in social skills. There may be discrepancies; intelligence may outstrip other areas and a bright child, promoted in school because of his advanced mental age may have adjustment difficulties because he is with a group of children who are physically and emotionally beyond him. Physical and psychological development depend upon both *hereditary* and *environmental factors*. Body development may be stunted, i.e. the child fails to reach his potential, because nutritional needs are not met, and if the environment fails to give the child adequate stimulation psychological stunting may occur. Socialization is the process through which the child comes to adopt attitudes and behaviour appropriate to the society in which he lives and is based primarily upon learning. Parents consciously teach good manners and how to behave in certain situations, but because of the child's inherent drive to imitate, much is learned from them without active teaching, including often, types of behaviour they would prefer the child not to copy. Although it relies heavily on animal studies, there is some evidence that during growth, *critical periods* occur when the environment must supply specific types of stimulation. If these are lacking, not only does development go astray but it is very difficult for the child to catch up if the needs are met at a later period. Thus, in the first three years, a child learns to trust others ('basic trust') if he receives consistent and affectionate parenting. If he does not, he may grow up handicapped by an inability to form satisfying emotional relationships.

## PERSONALITY

This relates to the distinguishing qualities of an individual which are displayed persistently in a wide variety of situations, especially social situations. It is the unique result of the interaction of the individual's genetic constitution and his environment. The child's personality has considerable potential for growth and change, in contrast to adults in whom personality traits are almost unalterable. Theories of personality development involve *intrinsic* factors (biological drives, hereditary

tempermental differences) and *extrinsic* (environmental) factors. Most
emphasise the effect of early childhood experience upon adult adjustment and behaviour. Two, are given in outline:

## Psychoanalytic theory

This is based on a conceptual framework developed by Freud and is
concerned essentially with emotional (psychosexual) development. Personality growth is seen as passing through a series of stages, each forming
a base for subsequent ones; thus firm foundations give a better chance of
a sound superstructure. If each is resolved successfully i.e. sufficient
emotional growth occurs to cope with stresses inherent to the individual
stage, the final result will be an adult who can work creatively, form
satisfactory interpersonal relationships and is unhampered by emotional
conflicts and anxiety. Difficulties at any stage can result in fixation or the
persistence of emotional conflicts apertaining to that stage. Although at an
unconscious level and the individual is unaware of what is troubling him,
these conflicts produce conscious anxiety, and behaviour, for which the
individual can give no rational explanation. Moreover, this anxiety
absorbs mental energy and reduces the personality's efficiency and chances
of satisfactory adjustment. If faced with stress, the individual tends to
regress to a stage at which he experienced difficulty and may show
behaviour appropriate to that stage. For example, if a child has a difficult
time as a toddler, a predisposition toward temper tantrums may persist
and infantile tantrums become very evident when he is faced with
difficulties at adolescence.

An important construct is an innate pleasure seeking drive, the *id*
whose focus changes during development, the focus being that area of the
body from which the individual obtains maximum pleasure at a given
stage. These stages of development are described as follows:

● *Oral stage* (first eighteen months). This is when maximum gratification
is obtained through oral activities; initially sucking, later biting and
chewing.

● *Anal stage* (eighteen months to three years), relates to a period when
interest shifts to excretory activities and gratification is obtained through
messiness and play with excretory products.

● *Phallic stage* (three years to six years) is characterised by the genitals
becoming the main source of pleasurable excitement. About this time, the
child develops an intense relationship with the parent of the opposite sex,
and hostile feelings toward the parent of the same sex (the Oedipal phase).

Difficulties relating to this are resolved by the process of identification with the parent of the same sex. The child realises he cannot usurp his father's place, so he attempts to become as like his father as possible.

● *Latency* (early school years). After the intense emotions of previous stages, a period of relative tranquillity occurs, this is the time when intellectual development forges ahead.

● *Genital stage* (puberty onwards). Gratification is now sought through adult-type sexual behaviour and eventually the development of a stable, heterosexual relationship.

In addition to the id which represents the basic drives or instincts, two other mental structures are described as functioning within the personality. These are the *ego*, or that part of the personality involved with interaction with the outside world, and the *superego*, or broadly speaking, the conscience. The ego's function is seen as mediating between reality, the superego and instinctual behaviour, allowing basic drives to be satisfied in a manner which is socially acceptable and consistent with the prohibitions of the superego.

These three parts of the personality form a dynamic system. Disturbance in one will upset the balance and produce readjustments in the others. If the superego is weak, the individual may get into trouble with society because his biological drives are satisfied in socially unacceptable ways. An abnormally strong superego will produce an individual who is excessively inhibited and guilt ridden and unable to satisfy his biological drives. Ego weakness may make the resolution of superego–id conflicts difficult or impossible.

## *Learning theory*

This is based on the premise that behaviour is modified by experience, and uses learning processes shown in animals to explain the shaping of human behaviour. It is concerned largely with the child and his social background. Differences in behaviour and attitudes are explained by the social rewards (approval) and punishments (disapproval) a child receives from parents, teachers and others in his environment when he exhibits different types of behaviour.

These two theories differ with regard to primary focus. Psychoanalytic theory is concerned with internal forces in the mind of the child, and social learning theory with the overt actions of the child. As a result, they are complementary rather than contradictory, and concepts derived from both may be of value in studying and understanding children.

## INTELLECTUAL DEVELOPMENT

Piaget's theory of cognitive development has also had an important influence on child psychology. The child is seen as developing increasingly complex patterns of thought and action, *mental schemata*, which are the basis of intelligence. This process starts at birth with simple reflexes and reaches full development in early adolescence with the ability to use formal logic. Mental schemata are developed by the processes of *assimilation* and *accommodation*. The first describes a process of taking in knowledge from the environment, which is then incorporated into the child's existing body of knowledge (in the same way as food is ingested and absorbed), the second a modification of existing knowledge by the new elements after they are taken in

Thus, to Piaget, intelligence is part of the process of adaptation of the organism to its environment and the environment must supply certain needs (*aliments*) for it to develop satisfactorily. Stages of development are:

● *Sensorimotor* (birth to about 18 months). During this period innate reflexes are modified and organised to become the elementary operations of intelligence so the child responds to stimuli in a meaningful way. Primitive mental imagery develops.

● *Pre-operational* (18 months to 7 years). The child begins to use mental symbols (images or words) and develops the ability to place objects in simple categories. Thought is dominated by his immediate perceptions (he often perceives only one aspect of an object or situation) and is egocentric i.e. he relates all observations to himself. Thus the sun and clouds are seen as following him around.

● *Concrete operations* (7 to 11 years). Mental processes become flexible and the child is able to focus on more than one aspect of a situation. Thought becomes reversible so he can return to the start of a mental operation if he wishes and repeat it. This gives him the ability to cope with the concept of number and complex classification of objects.

● *Formal operations* (11 to 13 years). The child is now able to use abstract concepts, to form and test hypotheses logically and his mental processes can operate entirely by the use of symbols.

Piaget stresses the vast difference between the thought processes of adult and child. Thus, in the pre-operational stage, the child is quite illogical. This has been demonstrated by a series of delightful experiments which anyone interested can easily repeat for themselves. A 4-year-old presented with equal quantities of liquid in identical glasses agrees they are equal, but insists they are different when the contents of one glass are poured into a tall, thin container, and the other into a wide, squat one. Because he can take into account only one dimension (the higher liquid level in the tall glass), this is regarded as having more in it. The child will cling to his belief in spite of the process being reversed and repeated in front of him. In the same way, equal quantities of dough rolled into balls are accepted as equal, but when their shapes are changed, then they are regarded as unequal. He is unable to grasp the principle of conservation, that quantity remains the same whatever the shape. Until 7 or 8, a child is quite oblivious of certain moral issues; thus a boy who is helping his mother and breaks fifteen cups is regarded as being more wicked than one who goes to a forbidden cupboard and breaks only one. The number of cups broken, and not motivation is seen as the basic issue. Piaget's ideas have been described in some detail in order to emphasise the need to attempt to see into the child's world. Those who work with children so often make the mistake of expecting the child to understand adult language and concepts, as for example when explaining a medical procedure to him.

## FOETAL DEVELOPMENT AND BIRTH

Factors which can influence a child's development are operative long before he achieves a separate existence and include:

### Physical events

These relate to the mother's health during pregnancy. Infections, ingestion of drugs and malnutrition (*Brit. Med. J.* 1976) may all affect the foetus, as may conditions such as placental insufficiency and antepartum haemorrhage, which reduce the oxygen supply to the developing brain.

## PSYCHOLOGICAL INFLUENCES

We know less about the effect of the mother's emotional state on the foetus than her physical condition. However, there is evidence from animal experiments and suggestive evidence from humans that severe or prolonged stress in the mother may affect foetal body size, adrenal size and levels of activity (Montagu 1962). Attitudes toward pregnancy are influenced by the mother's adjustment to her feminine role, the parenting she received and her relationship with the baby's father. Even in the most fortuitous circumstances many women are ambivalent toward their first pregnancy, doubting their adequacy and realising the big changes in life that having a child entails. The child may be perceived as a fulfilment and a means of perpetuating the admired traits of his forbears or in the case of an extramarital or unwanted pregnancy, an unwelcome nuisance. Anxieties relating to abnormality (physical and mental) in the child are almost universal and even today a surprising number of superstitious beliefs persist. Most women come to find their greatest fulfilment in bearing a child, but many have to work through some of the emotional aspects described above and may need help while they do this.

Animal studies show the need for the newly delivered mother to establish close physical contact with her offspring by licking and grooming; if opportunities for this are denied, the young may be rejected or even killed. Using as an analogy imprinting (a rapid process of irreversible learning which causes the young of some species to follow the parent figure), some writers suggest that the puerperium is a critical period for maternal-infant bonding and that maternity hospital conditions often mitigate against this (Klaus & Kennell 1976). As a result, hospital practice is allowing the infant to spend more time 'rooming in' with the mother than previously. If the baby is premature or 'delicate', he may be isolated from his mother for days or even weeks. Sometimes the mother is discharged home leaving him behind. Mothers whose infants have been separated from them in early days often complain of a feeling of the child not belonging to them.

## CHILDREN AND PARENTS DEVELOP TOGETHER

Developmental change in the child is reflected by changing attitudes in the parents. Some find it difficult to respond appropriately to the child's altering needs. A common failing is to treat him too much as a baby and hamper his steps toward independence.

*Infancy (year 1)* is the period of most rapid growth and transition from total dependence to a stage where the child is beginning to exert an influence on his environment. Specific features are:
● The establishment of *interpersonal relationships* within the family, starting with the mother. The development of the mother–child relationship is not a one way process but a steady interaction of two personalities, each calling out responses in the other. Social responses begin with a

smile as the mother is recognised at about 6 weeks of age and increase in complexity until by one year the child is playing simple games (pat-a-cake, peek-a-boo), obeying simple instructions and showing fear in response to strangers. Emotional responses gradually become differentiated, and by six months the child may experience and display pleasure, fear, anger and disgust.

● The establishment of satisfactory *physiological rhythms* in feeding, sleeping and elimination and learning to adjust these to a limited degree, to social demands.

● *Rapid motor development* which progresses through head control at three months, sitting at six months and standing with support at twelve months. Eye-hand co-ordination improves steadily and vocalisation increases rapidly in the second half of the period. By one year, isolated words may be recognisable.

● *Exploration of the environment* through eyes, ears, hands and mouth. There is a growing awareness of different parts of the body and of the self as a separate entity.

*The toddler stage ( year 2)* is characterized by:

● *Rapid motor development*, increasing mobility and physical independence. The child is into everything, exploring his environment at a prodigious rate. In spite of this physical independence, he lacks skill and judgement and limits must be set for his own safety (it is an age when accidents take a high toll of life and health), and this may lead to clashes with parental authority.

● This desire for *autonomy and self-assertiveness* often result in displays of *negativism*. The child learns the value of 'no' and 'won't' and uses them frequently. Frustration resulting in temper tantrums is common.

● The limitations set by parents eventually become an *internalised system of controls* forming the basis for conscience development.

● Reflex emptying of bladder and bowel gradually come *under voluntary control.* The child finds such activities pleasurable; he has no inhibitions about playing with excretory products and becomes keenly aware that his ability to hold on and perform in the wrong place can be used as a means of asserting himself. Normally he attempts to conform in order to please mother but if she is unduly strict and coercive, or lax and inconsistent in her approaches to toilet training, then soiling and wetting may persist after this stage.

● The bond between mother and child becomes intense and the child strongly *resists separation.* He clings to mother in strange surroundings or in the presence of strangers (stranger anxiety).

The parental tasks at this stage are to learn to set limits which allow for a reasonable degree of freedom, yet offer the child sufficient external controls to make him feel secure. Independence should be encouraged, but not at the expense of safety. Consistency in management is all important. Demands should be geared to what the child can reasonably be expected to achieve. The two year old's negativistic behaviour and temper tantrums should not be reciprocated by similar behaviour in the parents.

*Early childhood*, the pre-school period (years 3 to 5)
● There is a tremendous *growth in vocabulary* and constant chatter is characteristic as is intense curiosity. The child explores his environment continuously, often by persistent and repetitive questioning.
● *Fantasy* becomes an important part of the child's life; as his imagination grows 'tall stories' may worry parents. Fantasy playmates are common.
● Internal controls continue to develop by the *incorporation of parental attitudes*. Development of a sense of time enables the child to delay gratification in order to achieve his ends. He becomes more amenable to parental demands and co-operative with his family. A rudimentary conscience develops.
● Although still emotionally dependent upon parents, there is a *widening circle of social interaction*; with siblings at first, later with children in the neighbourhood or kindergarten. Co-operative patterns of play develop.

*The primary school child*
During this stage, the child gradually frees himself from infantile dependence on parents and learns the advantages and responsibilities of belonging to a peer group. He directs his energies to developing cognitive skills, and his interests widen tremendously.
● *Parents are no longer seen as omnipotent* as they were in the pre-school years. The school child questions their authority and expresses his individuality by attempting to make decisions for himself. In the early school grades, attitudes toward parents are transferred to teachers. If family relationships are satisfactory, then social adjustment to school is likely to be good.
● There is a steadily widening circle of *interpersonal relationships outside the family* as the child joins neighbourhood peer group activities such as Cubs or Brownies. He develops loyalties to these and learns the need to give and take in social interaction. Team games become very popular,

especially those involving rituals. Play is generally with children of the same sex.

● As thought processes become more flexible and the child is able to handle *abstract concepts*, he develops a scientific approach to his physical world, and continually experiments. Language becomes a useful tool both for the exchange of ideas and to influence others. Success in school will help the child learn to apply himself in order to achieve. Some children read voraciously.

● *Physical health* is generally good after immunity to common infections has been built up in the early school years. There is a great deal of energy to be dissipated, often in boisterous games. A considerable amount of time is spent in perfecting motor skills (skipping, swimming, riding a bicycle) and fine motor co-ordination (handicrafts, building models).

Parents must attempt to satisfy the child's curiosity and need for physical activity at this stage and allow him to develop individuality without becoming too eccentric. They must learn not to make unreasonable emotional demands upon him and to give him freedom to enjoy life with his peers.

The psychology of adolescence is described in Chapter 12.


## DEVELOPMENTAL ASSESSMENT

Early detection of children with handicaps, for example deafness or cerebral palsy, has, of course, important implications for management and training. Screening infants for irregularities in development is not difficult and requires only simple equipment. Three developmental screening tests are listed at the end of this chapter. In the very young child, diagnosis should not rest upon one observation but upon several, repeated over a period of time.


### References

BRITISH MEDICAL JOURNAL (1976) *Editorial*. The ultimate cost of malnutrition, **2**, 1158–59.
KLAUS M.H. & KENNELL J.H. (1976) *Maternal-infant Bonding*. St. Louis, C.V. Mosby Co.
MONTAGU M.F.A. (1962) *Prenatal Influences*. Springfield, Illinois. Thomas.

## General reading

HOWELLS J.G. Ed. (1965) *Modern Perspectives in Child Psychiatry.* London: Oliver & Boyd Ltd. Chapter 4 (Piagets theory). Chapter 6 (The application of learning theory to Child Psychiatry).
MUSSEN P. (1973) *The Psychological Development of the Child.* 2nd Ed. Englewood Cliffs N.J. Prentice Hall (A brief account of normal psychological development).
STONE L.J. & CHURCH J. (1973) *Childhood and Adolescence.* New York, Random House. Chapter 4 (Developmental principles and approaches).
TALBOT N.B., KAGAN J. & EISENBERG L. Eds. (1971) *Behavioural Science in Paediatric Medicine.* Philadelphia. W.B. Saunders Co. Chapter 4 (Children's learning). Chapter 7 (Personality development).

## Developmental screening tests

ILLINGWORTH R.S. (1973) *Basic Developmental Screening 0–2 years.* Oxford: Blackwell Scientific Publications.
KEMPE C.H., SILVER H.K. & O'BRIEN D. (1974) Denver developmental screening in *Current Paediatric Diagnosis and Treatment.* Oxford: Blackwell Scientific Publications.
SHERIDAN M. (1975) *The Developmental Progress of Infants and Young Children.* London: Her Majesty's Stationery Office.

# Chapter 3
# Psychopathology in Childhood

Mary, Mary, quite contrary
How does your garden grow?

Nursery Rhyme. Tom Thumb's
Pretty Song Book C 1744.

## EPIDEMIOLOGY. HOW COMMON IS
## PSYCHIATRIC DISORDER IN CHILDHOOD?

Studies relating to this should be evaluated critically remembering that:
● Children's behaviour can show wide variations and it is often hard to decide what is normal or abnormal for a given age.
● Many families fear that disturbed behaviour in a child reflects deficiencies in their management and are reluctant to draw attention to it.
● Parental tolerance toward certain types of behaviour in childhood such as restlessness, varies considerably.
● Cultural factors influence parents attitudes; thus Aboriginal or migrant families can have very different expectations for their children than other members of Australian society.
● Psychological disturbance in children may present with somatic symptoms or as a problem with schooling. These may be treated at face value and the underlying emotional disturbance go unrecognised.

### *Psychiatric disturbance in the primary school child*

Studies of children at this stage have shown that between 5 and 10% are 'maladjusted' i.e. show abnormalities of behaviour or emotional development.

If other conditions such as psychosomatic disorders and educational problems (which often require psychiatric help) are added, then the figure becomes considerably higher. One survey was carried out on the total population of children aged 10 to 11 years, resident in a circumscribed area, the Isle of Wight, in the U.K. (Rutter *et al.* 1970a). Defining psychiatric disorder as an abnormality of behaviour, emotions or interpersonal relationships sufficiently marked and prolonged to cause

37

persistent suffering or handicap to the child himself, and/or distress or disturbance in the family or community, a prevalence rate of 6.8% was found. This was regarded as a minimal estimate since uncomplicated intellectual handicap, educational retardation and isolated problems such as bed wetting were not included. This study showed that most disturbed children fitted into three groups:

1   *Neurotic disorders* which were characterised by symptoms of excessive anxiety and were commoner in girls.

2   *Conduct disorders*, characterised by antisocial behaviour. These were commoner in boys.

3   *Mixed conduct and neurotic disorders*. This group resembled group 2 in most characteristics but some evidence of neuroticism was present.

If 2 and 3 were pooled because of their similarities, the prevalence of neurotic disorder in the population studied was 2.5% and of conduct disorders 4.0%. The remaining 0.3% consisted of hyperkinetic disorders, psychosis and personality disorders (see p. 44).

## Psychiatric disturbance in early adolescence

The same population was re-examined when the children reached 14 to 15 years. The prevalence of psychiatric disorder had increased with age and was reported to be 21.0% (Rutter & Graham 1973). Although psycholoical disturbance increases around adolescence a threefold increase in four years is difficult to explain.

## Behavioural disturbance in pre-school children

Richman's (Richman *et al.* 1975) study of 3-year-old children living in London showed that 7% had behaviour problems rated moderate to severe and 15% had mild difficulties. There were no sex differences in frequency but boys were more likely to be overactive and show disturbances in sphincter control and girls more likely to show symptoms of 'nervousness'.

## Distribution of psychiatric disorder between the sexes

During primary school years, more boys than girls are referred for psychiatric help. This contrasts with adult psychiatric disturbance in which females predominate. Overall boys show a wider range of biological variation than girls and it has been suggested that they are more sensitive to environmental conditions as well (Rutter 1973). Since boys mature more slowly than girls, if their progress is compared with girls of the same age it may appear less favourable. Parents and teachers may be less tolerant of certain types of behaviour, e.g. aggressiveness, in boys.

### Specificity of symptoms

Most studies show significant differences between teachers and parents reports on a child's behaviour. A 'terrible problem' at school may not be evident at home and vice versa. This relates not only to the situational specificity of symptoms but to differences in perception of problem behaviour between parents and teachers.

### Childhood psychiatric disturbances in general practice

General practice surveys have shown that 10–20% of all patients are emotionally disturbed (Shepherd *et al.* 1966). Obviously the numbers reported will depend upon the orientation and discernment of the doctor and the population the practice serves. Figures relating to children are harder to obtain, but are probably of the same order, although families are increasingly turning to their general practitioner for help with behavioural problems. Since one traditionally visits a doctor with physical symptoms, many less vocal parents will utilise physical complaints as a means of communication.

A mother brought her seven-year-old girl with the complaint of recurring headaches. After three visits, it became obvious the child had experienced very little pain in her head or anywhere else. Her episodes of aggressive behaviour which the mother attributed to headaches, and the occasions when she 'screamed like mad' had raised serious worries that she had something 'pressing on her brain', like a grandparent who had died six months previously from a cerebral tumour. In fact, the 'attacks' showed a close relationship with the frequent parental quarrels which were disrupting the household, and the mother badly needed help with her marital problems.

*Do psychiatrically disturbed children receive help?*

The Isle of Wight study quoted above showed that only one in ten of the children with psychiatric disorder was under specialist psychiatric care. Others were being treated by family doctors or seeing probation officers or in residential schools for the maladjusted. Overall only one in five children with psychiatric disorder was having treatment. A similar situation was found in the young adolescents. Half the parents of these youngsters thought their child was disturbed, but most were unaware of services available. Middle class families tend to utilize child psychiatric services more than do those in poor socio-economic circumstances, yet follow-up studies show that the latter are more in need of help. When such families do reach a clinic, it is often because they have been forced to attend. This may prejudice the attitudes of both family and professional staff toward treatment.

## THE GENESIS OF PSYCHIATRIC DISORDER IN CHILDHOOD

The implications of finding aetiological factors are obvious. A summary of possibilities follows:
(Life situations commonly associated with childhood disturbance are described in Chapter 6.)

### Constitutional (hereditary) differences

Although a matter of some controversy it is generally held that intelligence is largely determined by genetic endowment, although a stimulating environment is still necessary for an individual to develop to his full potential. The extent to which personality traits are inherited is less certain. A longitudinal study by Thomas (Thomas & Chess 1976) has shown that babies display marked individual differences from birth and that these traits persist. It is easy to see how these could interact unfavourably with the environment to produce disturbance. For example an infant, by nature tense and irritable could fail to call out, loving responses in a mother whose personality traits make her sensitive to tension and who would establish a more satisfactory relationship if the child were placid.

## Physical injury and disease

Head injuries and infections, e.g. encephalitis, which are known to produce brain damage, may be followed by disturbed behaviour. Cerebral damage in the perinatal period is often blamed for behavioural disturbance. However, evidence is based often upon reports by parents whose response to a difficult child is to attempt to find a rational explanation and may be unreliable. Studies of premature babies and others at risk as regards perinatal cerebral insult have shown a higher percentage of behaviour problems than in normal controls. It must be remembered, that the anxiety of having a delicate child may influence parentel management and this could be responsible for the disturbance.

Rutter's study of the Isle of Wight school children (Rutter *et al.* 1970b) showed:

● A strong association between organic brain dysfunction (manifest by epilepsy or cerebral palsy) and psychiatric disorder. The prevalence of such disorder was 5 times that in the general population.

● That chronic physical disorder not involving the central nervous system e.g. asthma or deafness, was associated with psychiatric disturbance twice as commonly as in the general population.

Overall children with organic brain dysfunction showed psychiatric disturbance 3 times as commonly as children with chronic physical handicap. This suggests that the high rate of psychiatric disturbance in the first group was due to brain dysfunction itself, rather than being reactive to physical handicap, though the latter cannot be entirely excluded. Although the numbers were small, this study also confirmed the significant association between psychomotor epilepsy and psychiatric disorder, which has generally been reported in the literature (Graham & Rutter 1968).

## Parents attitudes

Children need dependable love, reasonable and consistent discipline and identity figures upon which to model their behaviour. If parents are unable to supply these, then, understandably character development may go astray. Obviously, his parents attitudes toward him will affect a child's self esteem. Kanner (1972) describes how parents attitudes (which relate to their own childhood experiences) can be envisaged as lying on a continuum between total acceptance (where the child is loved for what he is) and rejection (where the child is unwanted). A child may be rejected because his conception forced the parents into marriage, because he interrupted a career, was the wrong sex, resembles an unloved relative or was the result of an unplanned pregnancy, in which case he may be referred to as 'our mistake'. Three types of rejecting behaviour are described:

● *Overt hostility and neglect*, where the mother makes no attempt to establish a loving relationship. Children reared in this way show a shallowness of feeling and failure to respond to others emotionally. Aggressive behaviour and stealing are common features later.

● *Perfectionism*, where the mother, unable to face the guilt of not accepting a child rationalises that if he were tidier, more intelligent, physically different and so on, she could love him. Since no child can approach her standards of perfection, her excuse remains valid; moreover efforts to coerce him toward perfection give an excuse for punishment.

● *Compensatory overprotection*. The mother proves to herself, and the world, by her oversolicitude (smother love) that she is a good parent. She cannot give love so she gives excessive concern, food or material possessions in its place. It is not surprising that in the two latter situations, children become anxious and dependent or rebellious.

Fathers may collude with wives' attitudes. Some may compete for their wife's attention regarding their child as a rival; others may identify with the child and transfer deprecating or self-punishing attitudes to him. *Non-rejecting overprotection* may occur when a child is particularly precious, e.g. has survived a series of illnesses or is the only child of middle aged parents, and was conceived with difficulty. The parents' attitudes are understandable and do not indicate rejection and guilt. Nevertheless, help is needed in management, otherwise the child is at risk of becoming excessively infantilized.

## *Lack of mothering*

Bowlby's (1953) review of the effects of maternal deprivation in early life and his emphasis on the importance of attachment behaviour and the need for the child to form lasting bonds with adults, has been of very great value in drawing attention to the emotional needs of young children and to the often deplorable conditions which obtained in orphanages in the past. Recently, the concept has been reassessed by Rutter (Rutter 1972a), who suggests that experiences subsumed under the term 'maternal deprivation' are too heterogenous and its effects too varied for it to continue to have usefulness. Nevertheless animal studies (Harlow & Harlow 1969) show the need for parenting in primates. Studies of children reared in institutions and in foster homes (Skeels 1966) show thât for healthy mental development a young child needs a constant, parent figure (not necessarily his biological mother), who supplies sensory and emotional stimulation (talking and singing to him, carrying him around) as well as teaching the give and take necessary in close and affectionate relationships. To what extent the effects of maternal deprivation are reversible is uncertain but the longer the privation exists, the greater the chance of character defects developing (*Brit. Med. J.* 1976). Overell, research suggests that if the parent figure is:

● Completely absent, the infant's development may be seriously retarded physically, intellectually and socially. Subsequently, a cold affectionless psychopathic personality may develop.

● Present for a while, but later leaves the child, disrupting affectional bonds, the child becomes anxious, insecure and may show a variety of behaviour disturbances often antisocial in character.

● Present, but the quality of care is poor, because of the parents own personality difficulties, the child may show personality deviations resultant to this, and will often prove a poor parent in his turn.

## Absence of a father figure

The effect of this on the personality of boys has been studied (Biller 1970) and the following conclusions reached:

● *Impulsive and aggressive behaviour* are common. This seems to result from attempts to prove masculinity in a female dominated home and from lack of discipline.

● *Cognitive development suffers*, probably through lack of stimulation and because of social and economic difficulties. School work may be regarded as 'too feminine' since teachers, at least in early grades are usually female, and the boy rebels against it.

● There may be difficulties with *peer relationships* because of a lack of sex appropriate behaviour.

Obviously the mother's adequacy in filling a dual role, and the availability of adult male companionship outside the home is important. Andry (1971) among others, has shown a relationship between delinquency in boys and the lack of a father. A common finding is that the boy, seeking male company, becomes involved with a street gang whose behaviour is far from ideal.

# CLASSIFICATION OF CHILDHOOD PSYCHIATRIC DISORDERS – A MULTIAXIAL APPROACH

Disturbances of childhood are not easy to classify; growth and development may alter clinical features quickly and categories taken from adult psychiatric texts are not always appropriate. In 1967 the World Health Organisation attempted to develop 'a scientifically sound system of classification in child psychiatry' this was subsequently reviewed and revised (Rutter *et al.* 1975). The following is taken from that scheme:

## 0. Normal variation

The child's behaviour is compatible with normal variations in development.

## 1. Adaption reaction (reactive disorder)

Here the disturbance is outside the limits of normal, but there is no significant distortion of general development. These conditions are related to stress and are *transient* and *reversible*. Precipitating factors may be external, e.g. the loss of a parent, or internal, e.g. endocrine change at puberty.

## 2. Specific developmental disorders

These are specific delays or abnormalities in development which are related to biological maturation. One or several may be present in the same child. They are as follows:
  (i) Hyperkinetic disorder which is characterised by extreme over-activity, distractability, limited attention span and impulsivity.
 (ii) Speech and language disorders which are related to deficiencies in receptive or expressive language functions; often these co-exist. Articulatory disorders of speech (dyslalia) are also included.
(iii) Stammering (stuttering) in which there is a disorder of the rhythm of speech.
 (iv) Specific learning disorders which include specific reading retardation (dyslexia), specific retardation in arithmetic (developmental dyscalculia) and developmental perceptual disorders (these may be

in any modality but commonly relate to visual and auditory perceptual function).
(v) Abnormal clumsiness (developmental dyspraxia). The difficulties
may be in fine or gross motor co-ordination or both.
(vi) Enuresis ⎱ Failure to gain normal bladder or bowel control are
⎰ put into this category unless they are symptoms of some
(vii) Encopresis ⎰ other psychiatric disturbance or neurological disorder.
(viii) Tics (habit spasms). These are involuntary, apparently purposeless
and frequently repeated movements which are not due to any other
psychiatric or neurological condition.

### 3. Conduct disorder

*Conduct disorder* is used for abnormal behaviour which gives rise to social
disapproval. Some of these children may be delinquent, i.e. are in, or are
likely to be in contact with the law, but other types of behaviour such as
bullying and fighting may be included.

### 4. Neurotic disorder

*Neurotic disorder* is used to describe conditions where there are abnormalities of feeling and behaviour but these are not accompanied by a loss of
reality sense (as in psychosis). Into this category come states of anxiety or
depression disproportionate to environmental events. Obsessions, compulsions, phobias, hypochondriasis and conversion reactions are also
included. For amplification and explanation of these terms see p. 103–8.

### 5. Personality disorder

This category is used for individuals who show long-standing, relatively
fixed abnormalities of behaviour. It is not commonly applied in early and
middle childhood, but reserved for older children and adolescents, in
whom more persistent behaviour patterns may be shown.

### 6. Psychoses

These are mental disturbances in which the individual shows severely
disturbed, bizarre and unpredictable behaviour. Much has to be learned

about childhood psychosis, but for the present the following sub-
categories are used:

(i) Infantile psychosis, which begins in the first 3 years of life.

(ii) Late onset psychosis. This occurs after a period of normal development and generally after the age of 4–6 years. Because this involves
profound regression and often a loss of speech and other functions,
the term disintegrative psychosis is sometimes used.

(iii) Adult-type psychoses seen in older children. Schizophrenia-like
illness, and very rarely, manic-depressive psychosis may occur.

(iv) Other types, for example where a child comes to accept the false
beliefs (delusions) of a psychotic relative and 'folie - deux' develops.

## 7. *Psychosomatic disorders*

These are disorders with organic pathology in which psychological factors
play a major role in aetiology.

## 8. *Manifestations of mental subnormality.*

## 9. *Other clinical syndromes*

This category includes acute and chronic brain syndromes, i.e. cases
where organic brain impairment is evident. These may be acute and
transitory, e.g. following drug ingestion, or chronic and irreversible, e.g.
following head injury or encephalitis. Anorexia nervosa (see p. 205) and
Tic de Gilles de la Tourette (see p. 155) are also included.

Disorders of eating and sleeping, and habit disorders, such as nail
biting, thumb sucking and head banging are not included in this classification. These are not regarded as psychiatric abnormalities if they occur in
isolation, and when they occur as part of another disorder they should be
placed with that in the classification scheme.

Because of the importance of the child's intellectual level and other
aetiological factors in the overall assessment of a case a *multiaxial classification is* suggested:

*Axis one:* The clinical psychiatric syndrome. A category from the
classification above. This is essentially descriptive in nature.

*Axis two:* Intellectual level. This is assessed clinically. Often psychometric assessment by a psychologist is used.

*Axes three and four:* These relate to biological, psychological and social influences which contribute to a child's disturbance. Axis three involves physical factors, axis four psychosocial.

## The case formulation

This is a valuable method of summarising the many variables which need to be considered when assessing a disturbed child. A formulation should include:
1. Name, age and sex of child.
2. Presenting symptoms.
3. Diagnosis – includes axes one and two.
4. Aetiology – axes three and four.
5. Further investigations.
6. Treatment plan.
7. Prognosis.

For example: Peter, a 9-year-old boy, presented with complaints of stealing from local shops. This behaviour is one aspect of the conduct disorder from which he suffers. He is of dull normal intelligence. The aetiology of his condition relates to the absence of a father figure (father is in gaol), lack of supervision by mother, who is in whole time employment, extremely poor housing conditions, and the example set by an older brother. Further investigations include a home visit by the social worker to assess the help grandparents can give, and a school report on his educational achievement. Treatment will be directed toward helping the mother with her pressing social problems, advising on management, and involving the patient in youth club activities. In view of the multitude of problems this family faces the prognosis should be guarded.

## THE RELATIONSHIP BETWEEN CHILD AND ADULT PSYCHIATRIC DISORDER

This has most important implications for the organisation of Child Psychiatric Services and may be approached in two ways:
1. By long term follow-up of disturbed children.
2. By retrospective studies of adult psychiatric patients.
Difficulties are inherent in both. The long periods of time involved, changes in diagnostic categories over the years and the mobility of families in Australia today, are obvious ones.

## Psychopathy

Robins (1966) follow up of child guidance clinic patients showed that about one half who presented with delinquent behaviour became adult psychopaths. Case histories of psychopathic adults confirms this. Most show evidence of antisocial traits dating from at least late childhood. We do not know however, what makes these traits persist, but there is a strong suggestion that environmental factors are important. Slater (1953) showed that both monozygotic and dizygotic twins showed a high level of concordance for sociopathy. Bohman quoted by Rutter (1972b) showed that criminality in parents was not associated with antisocial behaviour in their offspring if the latter were placed for adoption in infancy. However, if these children were reared by their natural parents then their antisocial rating was high.

Attention has recently been paid to the follow-up of children with minimal brain dysfunction (see p. 165). Menkes (Menkes *et al.* 1967) reported that as adults, many show poor social adjustment; antisocial traits and criminal behaviour are not uncommon and a few become psychotic.

## Other psychiatric syndromes

'Neurotic traits of childhood' viz. nail biting, bed-wetting, stammering – beloved of adult psychiatric texts – are not neurotic nor are they associated with neurotic illness in later life. A minority of children with symptoms resembling those of neurosis in adult life such as excessive anxiety, phobias and obsessions do persist with these traits, but most children labelled neurotic do not become neurotic adults, although there is a higher incidence of non-specific psychiatric abnormality among them than among normal controls when adulthood is reached (Robins 1966).

Depressive illness is being recognised with increasing frequency in childhood but its relation to adult depressive disorders has to be defined. Nevertheless it seems likely that sensitization to loss (often of a parent figure) in childhood may be a precursor of depression in later life. There is probably no relationship between infantile autism and schizophrenia but a psychiatric disturbance resembling schizophrenia as it is manifest in adults may occur in later childhood (see Chapter 10). Indeed with the approach of adolescence, clinical syndromes resembling, but in general less well differentiated, than in adults, may be recognised. 'Adolescent turmoil' has been used to describe an acute behavioural disturbance believed to be reactive to stress in adolescence but there appears to be no specificity about it and in general, disturbances in adolescence fall into four areas; mild emotional disorder from which the youngster emerges unscathed, neurosis which carries a good prognosis, sociopathy which has a much less favourable outcome and schizophrenia which does worst of all.

Mellsop's (1972) study of over 3,000 disturbed children seen in a Melbourne hospital, showed that three and one-third times as many as would be expected in the normal course of events, became patients of the State Adult Psychiatric Department in later life. As found in previous studies, children showing reactions to environmental stress had the best prognosis; males with sociopathic traits the worst.

## References

ANDREY R. (1971) *Deliquency and Parental Pathology*. London, Staples Press.
BILLER H.B. (1970) Father absence and personality development in the male child. *Developmental Psychol.* 2, 2, 181–201. (*Annual Progress*, Vol. 4, 1971).
BOWLBY J. (1953) *Child Care and the Growth of Love*. Ed. M. Fry. Ringwood, Victoria: Penguin Books Australia Ltd.
BRITISH MEDICAL JOURNAL (1976) *Editorial*, Koluchova's twins, 2, 897–898.
GRAHAM P. & RUTTER M. (1968) Organic brain dysfunction and child psychiatric disorder. *Brit. Med. J.*, 3, 695–700. (*Annual Progress*, Vol. 2, 1969).
HARLOW H.F. & HARLOW M.K. (1969) Effects of various mother-infant relationships on rhesus monkeys behaviours in B.F. Foss (ed) *Determinants of Infant Behaviour*, Vol. 4, London, Methuen.
KANNER L. (1972) *Child Psychiatry* (4th ed). Springfield, Illinois, Charles C. Thomas. Chapter 9.
MELLSOP G.W. (1972) Psychiatric patients seen as children and adults: childhood predictors of adult illness. *J. Child Psychol. and Psychiat.* 13, 91–101. (*Annual Progress*, Vol. 6, 1973).
MENKES M., ROWE J.S. & MENKES J.H. (1967) A 25 year follow-up study on the hyperkinetic child with minimal brain dysfunction. *Paediatrics*, 39, 393–399.
RICHMAN N., STEVENSON J.E. & GRAHAM P.J. (1975) Prevalence of behaviour problems in 3-year-old children: an epidemiological study in a London borough. *J. Child Psychol. and Psychiat.* 16, 277–287.
ROBINS L.N. (1966) *Deviant Children Grown Up*. Baltimore, Williams and Wilkins.
RUTTER M., TIZARD J. & WHITMORE K. (1970a) *Education, Health and Behaviour*. 178–201. London, Longmans.
RUTTER M., GRAHAM P.J. & YULE W. (1970b) *A Neuropsychiatric Study in Childhood*. Clinics in Developmental Medicine No. 35/36. London, Spastics International Medical Publications with Heinemann.
RUTTER M. (1972a) *Maternal Deprivation Reassessed*. Ringwood, Victoria, Penguin Books Australia Ltd.
RUTTER M. (1972b) Relationships between adult and child psychiatric disorder. *Acta Psychiatrica Scandinavica*, 48, 3–21. (*Annual Progress*, Vol. 6, 1973).

RUTTER M. & GRAHAM P. (1973). Psychiatric disorder in the young adolescent:
a follow-up study. *Proc. Roy. Soc. Med.* **66**, 1226–1228.
RUTTER M. (1973) *Helping Troubled Children.* Pp. 103–108. Ringwood Victoria.
Penguin Books Australia Ltd.
RUTTER M., SHAFFER D. & SHEPHERD M. (1975) *A Multi-axial Classification of
Child Psychiatric Disorders.* An evaluation of a Proposal. Geneva, World
Health Organisation.
SHEPHERD M., COOPER B., BROWN A.C. & HILL I.D. (1966) *Psychiatric Illness in
General Practice.* London, Oxford University Press.
SKEELES H.M. (1966) Adult status of children with contrasting early life ex-
periences. *Monogr. Soc. Res. Child Dev.* Vol. 31.
SLATER E.T.O. (1953) *Psychotic and Neurotic Illness in Twins.* London, H.M.S.O.
THOMAS A. & CHESS S. (1976) *Temperament and Development.* New York,
Brunner/Mazel.
* See Appendix B.

# Chapter 4

# The Case History: Assessment of the Child

'Begin at the beginning' the king said, gravely
and go on till you come to the end: then stop.'
Lewis Carroll (Charles Lutwidge Dodgson) 1832-1898.
*Alice in Wonderland.*

Taking a history is an important step in helping the disturbed child and his family. The child psychiatrist has few laboratory aids and is dependent on information obtained from history taking and his observation of the child in making a diagnosis. Graham and Rutter (1968) have shown that information derived from psychiatric interviews with parents and with children is both valid and reliable.

Whether the parents are seen separately, or together with the child depends upon the individual case. The nature of the problem, the age of the child, and the experience of the interviewer are all considerations. Seeing a family together can be very helpful but is demanding for the person who conducts the interview, and many beginners in child psychiatry prefer to see child and parents separately. If this is the case, how they separate should be noted. Sometimes a mother clings to her child anxiously or tells the staff how badly behaved he will be in her absence. The child may be very distressed at the prospect of leaving his parents. If this happens, it is best not to enforce separation but see child and parents together briefly and having shown the child that he will be neither reprimanded nor kept at the clinic (both of which may have been suggested to him), arrange for later visits when he can be seen alone.

Older children can be very suspicious of what is being said in their absence, feeling that the doctor is siding with their parents. If this is likely to be the case it is better to see the child first, or to arrange for the parents and the child to visit the clinic separately. When talking to the child, it is reasonable to inform him that his parents will be seen, but it may be necessary to stress the confidentiality of the doctor–patient relationship and to explain that information given by him will not be divulged to his parents, unless he wishes. When such a promise is given, it must never be broken.

Some clinics arrange for a preliminary history to be taken by a social worker before the family visits the clinic. This has the advantage of the

psychiatrist knowing something about the patient's background before he
sees the family, and the disadvantage that preconceived ideas on the part
of parents and psychiatrist may affect interaction when they finally meet.
Probably this procedure is best restricted to cases which, on initial referral,
appear to be basically social problems likely to need social worker
involvement.


## INTERVIEW WITH THE PARENTS

The aim should be quiet surroundings and lack of interruptions. Younger
siblings are best excluded. They are distracting and parents may divert
attention to them as a means of evading difficult subjects. 'Don't touch
that switch Johnny', will always distract the examiner. Siblings may give
a garbled account of happenings to the patient later. Both parents must
be seen whenever possible, together initially, but separate interviews may
be necessary subsequently. Whoever is conducting the interview should
make his identity clear at the start. The numbers of staff met in clinic or
hospital can be bewildering and people wish to know to whom they are
divulging information.


### The function of the interview

This can be therapeutic as well as fact finding. Parents may come after
months of anxiety and condemnation by others for the child's misdeeds;
finding an authority figure who can listen and accept what they say without
criticism can be a great relief. As they discuss their worries, tension eases
and they see the problem more objectively; because of this, symptoms
often improve after the first visit.


### Allocation of time

At least an hour is needed for an adequate history and this should be
allowed for in the appointment book. If it seems likely that more time than
this will be necessary, parents should be warned that the interview will
have to be terminated and advised that another will be arranged at a later

date. It is realised that much of what is said in this chapter could be difficult to achieve in general practice. However, the family doctor starts with the advantage of knowing the background from which the patient comes and it is not impossible for an interested doctor to allow wider spacing of appointments for some sessions.

## Note taking

Interviews of this length usually need recording as they go, however the act of writing should not be allowed to detract from the examiner's efficiency as an observer. Rough notes, which can be organised later, are probably best until the examiner evolves his own technique. Sometimes audio-visual recordings are made. These should never be done without the parents' consent.

## Interaction during the interview

The relationship which develops between the examiner and parents on the first occasion they meet will form a basis for subsequent interactions, and should be given the respect it deserves. If the interviewer can establish his role as a sympathetic, interested listener who encourages parents to tell their own story, then satisfactory rapport will be achieved. A list of quick-fire direct questions will elicit quick-fire direct answers, and little else. At the end of a 'fact-finding' interview, the student may find himself with a mass of facts, but little comprehension of what is really happening in the child's life. Face-saving should be allowed by the questioner assuming negatively valued behaviour. 'Do you hit your child ?' will usually produce a negative answer. 'How often do you find it necessary to punish him ?' a truthful response.

Attention must be paid to *non-verbal* as well as *verbal communication*. The tone of voice, the physical concomitants of emotion – a trembling hand or the suspicion of tears – will indicate areas of particular sensitivity. It is often wise to follow such observations up. 'Why is this so worrying for you ?' or 'that seems to matter a lot'. Not only will this reveal information, but rapport will be strengthened as the parents feel the interviewer is sensitive to their anxiety without them being forced to raise an issue. If a particular subject seems very painful, it may be wise to leave it for another time. Pushing too hard may result in never seeing the parents again.

## Developing insight

Students must remember that their attitudes to parents and children may relate to their own childhood experiences. If one finds one's self unreasonably angry or unduly sympathetic to a certain situation, it is wise to discuss these feelings with the supervisor of the case and attempt to discover why this has happened. A degree of detachment is necessary in order to function efficiently, but this should not lead to impersonal handling of families. Most people try to be good parents and are sensitive about their failings. Condemnation by the examiner has no place in the management of disturbed families.

## Structure of the interview

The student should not allow himself to be sidetracked into a discussion of the parents' personal difficulties unless they are important to the child. A firm reminder that the purpose of the interview is to discuss the child's problems may be necessary.

The aim should be to achieve a *balance between flexibility* (allowing parents to express themselves freely) and *keeping to a scheme* which ensures adequate fact finding. With this in mind, the following scheme is suggested:

1 *Informant* and his/her relationship to the child. *Agency* referring the case.

2 *Age*, school and grade.

3 The parents should be asked to state what their *complaint* is in their own words (this often differs significantly from the referring letter).

4 *History of present difficulties.* This is what the parents have come about, understandably they want to talk about it first. Occasional questions may be necessary or an example asked for, but in general, parents should be allowed to present the problem as they see it. When they finish, enquiry should be made as to the presence of other symptoms indicating behavioural, emotional or intellectual difficulties, or evidence of psychosomatic disorder.

5 *Family:*

(i) Parent figures. Whether natural parents, step-parents or adoptive.

(ii) Other adults in the house, e.g. grandparents.

(iii) Child's position in family. Ages of siblings.

(iv) Social background. Occupation and educational status of parents.

(v) Estimate of the emotional climate of the home, e.g. happy or disturbed due to constant bickering between the parents.

(vi) Health of family members, both physical and psychiatric.

6 *Developmental history:*

(i) Pregnancy, birth, and early months. Enquiry should be made as to any events which could have affected central nervous system development, e.g. hypoxia in the perinatal period or infection. Psychological aspects of the pregnancy must not be neglected. It is important to know whether the child was wanted and planned, and was the sex which the parents wanted. Tactful enquiry will reveal whether the conception was premarital, and even the reason for the parents marrying at all. 'Had you been married long before John (the patient) arrived ?' is the best way of putting this.

(ii) Rate of passing developmental milestones. Basically these are:

Age of first social response—smiling.

Age when first sat up (alone and not propped).

Age of taking first steps without support.

Age of achieving habit training, such as bowel and bladder control.

Speech development. Age of babbling. Age when first recognisable words (not dad-dad or mum-mum) were used appropriately. Age when word linkage occurred.

Many mothers cannot remember specific details; asking them how the child's development compared with his normal siblings (or children living nearby) will usually give a good indication of whether the child's rate of development lies within normal limits.

(iii) First reactions to kindergarten and/or school.

7 *School.* Enquiry should be directed toward:

(i) Academic achievement.

(ii) Social adjustment.

A teacher's report can be invaluable, providing an objective account of the child's progress and of his interaction with authority figures and with his peers. A request for a report will often be the start of a cooperative relationship between doctor and teacher which can be of great benefit to the child.

8 *Medical history.* It is important to know not only about any physical illness which the child has suffered, but how he and his family reacted to it, and what family attitudes are toward illness generally.

9 *Conclusion.* As the interview ends and satisfactory rapport has been established, it is worthwhile asking the parents what they feel has produced their child's disturbance. It is surprising how much insight parents

can develop while talking through their difficulties with a sympathetic advisor and this may be used as a start toward helping them.

*Writing up notes*

Students are often bewildered by the mass of information they obtain when taking a psychiatric history. Organisation is essential if full use is to be made of it. Temporal relationships can often be clarified by constructing a chart of events happening within the family. An example is given here in table 4.1:

TABLE 4.1

| YEAR | FATHER | MOTHER | PATIENT | SIBLING 1 | SIBLING 2 |
|---|---|---|---|---|---|
| March | Accident at work. Hospitalised | Anxiety symptoms visits doctor, tranquilliser prescribed· | | | |
| April | | | Nightmares develop | Starts wetting the bed | |
| May | Returns home | Still on tran- quillisers, but improved | | | |
| June | | Off tablets | | | |
| July | Returns to work | | Sleeping well | Occasional wet bed | |
| August | | Grandmother visits home, incessant arguments over childrens' management | Nightmares recur | Dry at night | School re- fusal, visits clinic |
| Sept. | | Grandmother leaves | Still sleeping poorly | | Referred for remedial help at school, goes to school happily |
| Oct. | | | Sleep improved | | |

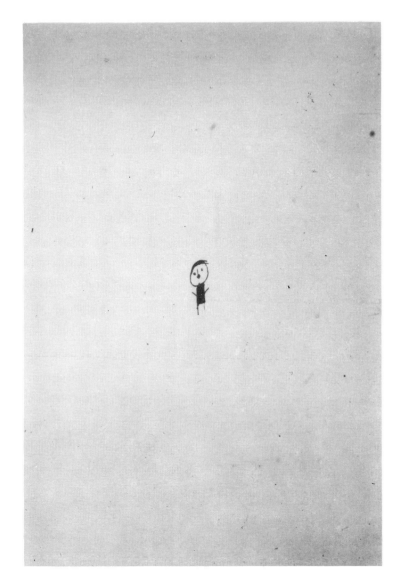

FIGURE 4.1. This picture of himself was drawn by a 6-year-old boy of exceptionally small stature. The aetiology of his condition was unknown. Although of normal intelligence he had been kept down a grade at school because of his physical dimensions. He was very angry about this and started to steal and to damage the belongings of adults in his family circle. When he buried the contents of his father's tool box all over the garden, the situation reached a climax and help was sought. Friends and family members were portrayed together using most of the paper. He refused to include himself in these composite pictures and continually produced this tiny figure standing alone, leaving the rest of the page quite empty when asked to draw himself.

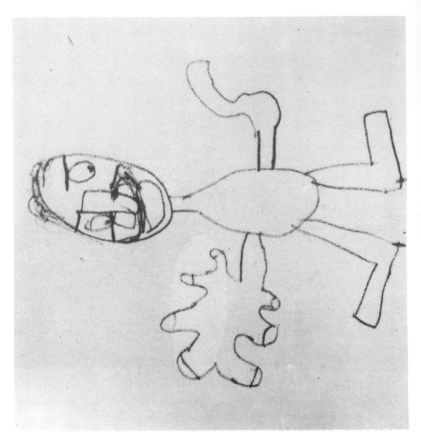

FIGURE 4.2. This picture of 'my dad' was drawn by an 8-year-old boy referred because of school difficulties. He had a severe auditory perceptual problem and was quite unable to carry out the complicated messages his father shouted at him. His father was known to physically abuse him under the guise of punishment, and a younger sibling had been admitted to hospital as a 'battered child' with two broken arms. The father's hypertrophied right hand suggests the significance it had for the patient, and how often it had been applied to his gluteal region.

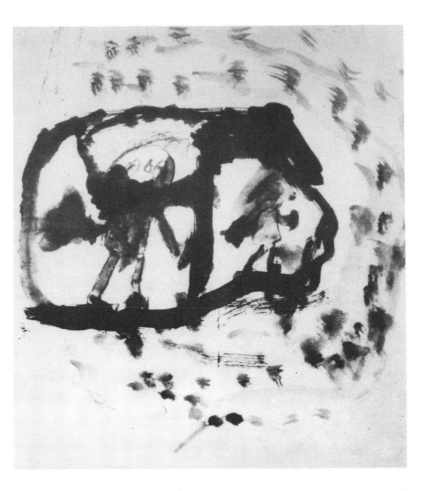

FIGURE 4.3. A painting by an asthmatic child, depicting her recent hospital admission. She is the figure on the left. The black, constricting bands which surround her and cover her mouth are an attempt to show 'how she felt'. They even involve the nurse, the figure on the right who is coming to help her.

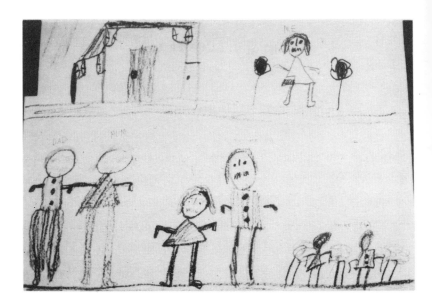

FIGURE 4.4 and 4.5. Like figure 4.3, these are also produced by an asthmatic child, an 8-year-old girl who shows herself at home and in hospital. Figure 4.4 shows her home and family. It is colourful, involves the use of the whole page. Her only adverse comment was that her twin siblings, of whom she was very jealous and who are shown by small figures in the extreme right hand corner, had got lost in the wood. Figure 4.5, shows her in hospital. The whole picture was executed in blue and purple, giving it a cyanotic effect. She said how lonely and empty the ward was. Note the emptiness of the paper.

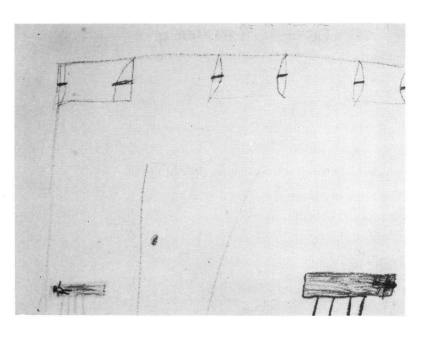

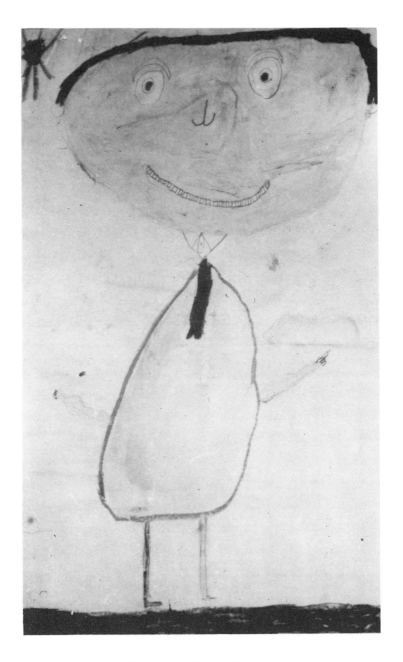

FIGURE 4.6. A picture of 'my doctor' by a child who had undergone repeated surgery for congenital malformations. The doctor has over 30 teeth and a right arm shaped like a hypodermic.

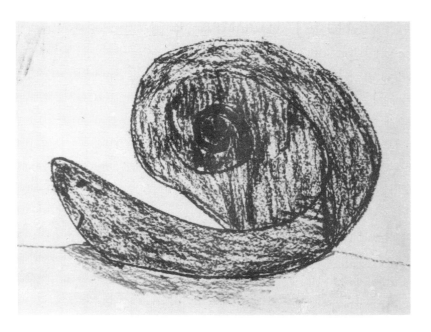

FIGURE 4.7. A picture of 'how I feel' by a 9-year-old boy who suffered from both chronic constipation and a mother who focused family attention on the state of his bowels. It was hardly surprising that it was executed in brown crayon.

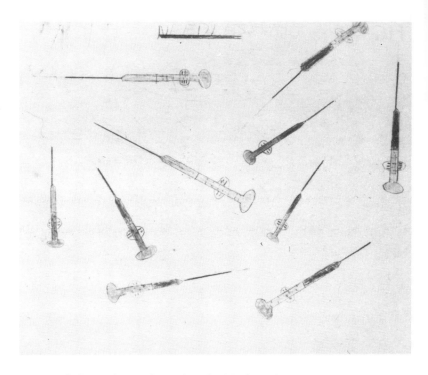

FIGURE 4.8. Drawn by another asthmatic girl of 11 who had a history of repeated admissions to hospital. As an exercise at school she was asked to demonstrate what the word 'hospital' meant to her. She was a timid, reserved child whose high level of anxiety was noted whenever she visited hospital.

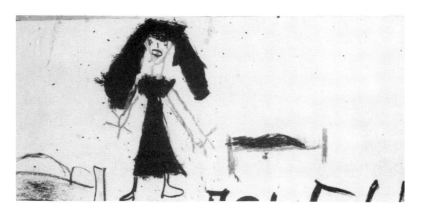

FIGURE 4.9. A group of children in a hospital school were asked to portray hospital scenes. This is an example of a very common theme, 'a nurse taking blood'. Mostly the nurses were coloured red, although in fact the standard uniform was white. In this particular example, the vampire like creature had red hair as well as red garments. Her left arm also has hypodermic characteristics. When questioned about their reasons for drawing this subject, the children were unanimous in saying they hated it most, if was scary. When questioned as to what they thought the staff did with the blood, most became very defensive, but one small boy reported that he felt 'weak and poisoned' afterwards.

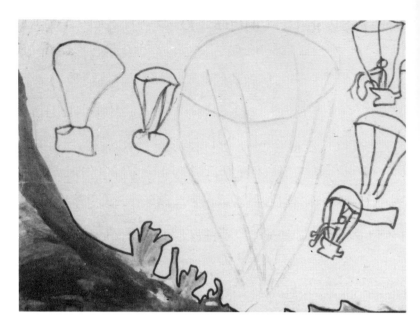

FIGURE 4.10. This is a glimpse into the bizarre world of the psychotic child. This boy who is described in Chapter 10 drew parachutists descending from a plane. Two of them are sitting on toilets.

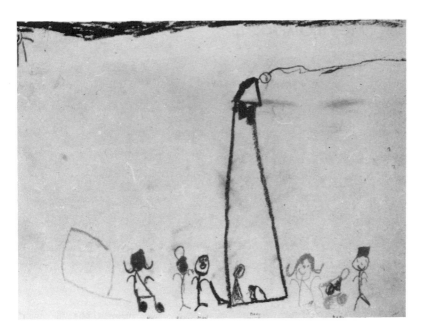

FIGURE 4.11. This 4½-year-old girl had suffered severe physical abuse and a vaginal tear as the result of an attack by a 'friend' of her father. Psychiatric assessment was requested as she remained quite mute after several days in hospital. On entering the offices, she was asked to portray her home and family Figure 4.11. This she did quite quickly and silently. The tall object is her home. The figure standing immediately to the left of the house was drawn in black, in contrast to the others which were portrayed in colour. When questioned as to who this was, she suddenly found her voice, 'He's a bad man with a stick that he stuck in my tummy'. She then named the other figures who were members of her family, but returned to the black figure again and again, and expressed verbally some of the aggression she felt about the assault. This formed the starting point of verbal communication between the child and the writer, who was able to reassure her that care would be taken of her in the future. After this episode she spoke normally again.

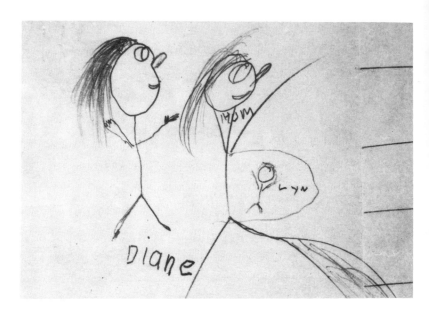

FIGURE 4.12. A 7-year-old girl from an emotionally deprived background came into hospital following a series of accidents and illnesses. She produced this picture during an art session in the hospital school. When asked if the small figure within the mother's abdomen was a new baby, she said, 'No, that's me, I'm back where it is safe and bad things can't happen.'

When he has thought over the interview and completed his notes, the student should consider carefully:

● The type and extent of the child's disturbance. Is further information necessary, e.g. a school report?

● The parents' motives in bringing the child. Do they really want help for themselves or for the child? Do they wish the child's management to be taken over from them or do they even want him out of the home?

Further interviews may be necessary to explore details, but the basic information necessary to plan treatment can be obtained at the first encounter in most cases.

## INTERVIEW WITH THE CHILD

Communicating with children can be a fascinating experience, as students who take the trouble to talk to children will learn. Children can give a good account of themselves and their background, but it takes time and patience to establish a satisfactory relationship which allows them to do so. An introduction is important. Children are generally more confused than parents as to the identities of personnel. They should be informed clearly of the examiner's name and role. Clinics have strong associations with hypodermics in the minds of most young children, and reassurance may be necessary. A few minutes spent discussing superficial topics will enable the child to assess the examiner and the situation, and will reduce his anxiety level. The interview rooms does not need elaborate equipment; a few toys appropriate to the child's age, and paper and coloured crayons are sufficient. Quietness and absence of interruptions are as important as when seeing the parents. Whether the examiner sits behind a desk is a matter of preference. Some feel that it separates the examiner from his patient, or resembles the school situation too closely and avoid it. Note taking may distract the child's attention or make him suspicious. If necessary, the purpose, and the confidential nature of anything said by the child should be explained.

### *Methods of communication*

The younger the child the less is he able to express himself in words, and the more important do non-verbal methods of communication become. Play can be utilized as a means of expression. A doll's house with figures representing father, mother, boy child, girl child and baby presented to a child under about 6 years will contribute to an understanding of family dynamics. It does not require much perspicacity to interpret the meaning of father and mother figures placed in separate beds at opposite ends of the house, or of the baby doll being pushed head first into the toilet. Both have been observed in the author's clinic.

Children's paintings and drawings can also be informative, especially a request to portray home and family. While the child's attention is absorbed with drawing and defences less active, he will produce more information than if he were fixed on a chair and staring at the examiner.

*Helping children to talk*

Questions addressed to the child must be at a level appropriate to his comprehension. It is useless expecting children to understand adult language, and worse still medical jargon. Some workers respond intuitively to the child's answers, phrasing their next question more appropriately. However, many students find it difficult to gear communication to the child's level. Only experience with children will teach what is and is not appropriate. It is equally embarrassing for older children to be treated in an infantile way as it is for the young child to be asked incomprehensible questions. To discuss one's difficulties with an adult is not a natural way of behaving in childhood. Remember the child has not come to the clinic of his own accord, in fact, he was probably most reluctant to do so. Why should he tell a complete stranger about his private thoughts?

Sometimes it is a help to ask him why he came; his reply may be startling and reflect his parents' methods of persuading him to come. If he is unable or unwilling to answer this, the parents' stated reason for bringing him may be given, and his opinion sought on this matter.

Instead of discussing their problems directly, some young children find it easier to tell *their story in the third person*, about a child of their age and sex. Generally it becomes translated into the first person as the interview progresses. Other ways of seeing into the child's world are to enquire about his dreams and fantasies. The time-honoured method of *asking for three wishes* is quite useful for the child under nine years or so. One child with a severe reading disability showed preoccupation with school failure by saying:
'I wish the school bus broke down.'
'I wish the school was burned down.'
'I wish the teacher was dead.'

*Once adequate rapport is established*, even simple questions may produce a wealth of information. For example, a six-year-old boy replying to a standard intelligence test question, 'What comes in a bottle ?', said 'Plonk, wine, metho, and beer', and as an afterthought, 'shampoo'. A social worker subsequently confirmed heavy drinking by both parents.

A six-year-old girl rejected by her parents in favour of two brighter siblings drew her recent birthday party. She produced figures representing her family but not herself. When questioned, she replied, 'I wasn't there. Mummy and Daddy wouldn't let me come.'

## In summary

Communication with the child under five years is best established through play and drawing or finger painting; between five and eight years through painting and telling stories; after eight years, verbal communication becomes easier with less emphasis being placed on other methods, although with a very inhibited child they may be necessary.

## What can be learned from the interview?

The examiner should learn from the older child:

1　His attitudes toward the problems which have brought him to the clinic.
2　His attitudes towards members of his family.
3　His feelings about school; both from the academic point of view and how he gets along with other children.
4　His interests and hobbies and how he relates generally to significant people in his environment.
5　Whether he has overwhelming worries or anxieties; his attitudes to somatic symptoms if these are present. Whether he has experienced any abnormal mental phenomena such as hallucinations.

Whatever the age of the child the examiner should also assess:

1　*Appearance*. Dress and physical development in relation to age should be noted, also characteristics which might make the child stand out from his peers.
2　*Motor development*. Whether the child is hyper- or hypoactive; well or poorly coordinated; left or right handed.
3　*Attention span*. Can the child concentrate on a task or is he restless and distractable.

4 *Speech.* Both articulation (motor development) and ability to use words (language development).

5 *Manner of relating.* This will give a good indication of relationships with other adults in the environment. The child may be friendly and trusting, sullen and resentful, or sometimes highly manipulative.

6 *Level of intelligence.* If old enough to attend school, grade in relation to age will give an indication. In general, verbal ability correlates with intelligence as does a long list of interests, hobbies and activities. Some workers ask questions from one of the standard intelligence tests (e.g. the W.I.S.C.), or assess the child on his ability to draw a human figure (Goodenough-Harris Draw-*b*-Man Test). Both these tests are described in Chapter 5. Questions involving general knowledge can be useful, but the examiner must know what is appropriate for a given age, and make allowance for environmental factors.

7 *Emotional state.* Whether the child's anxiety is inappropriate to the situation. Whether he is cheerful and confident, or predominantly unhappy.

*Physical examination* is an important part of the diagnostic process and should generally be done at the first interview. Although some psychiatrists prefer to refer the child for assessment by a paediatrician, this is generally unnecessary. A physical examination is expected by the child when he visits the doctor and helps him understand the doctor is interested in his total functioning.

As the interview ends, any *further investigations* planned for example, psychological assessment, should be explained to the patient. A brief discussion of the nature of the child's symptoms and plans for treatment is worthwhile if it is within the limits of the child's comprehension.

It is often not possible to obtain all this information during one interview. Students must be prepared to build up a picture of the child over several sessions. Rigid questioning and conformity to an 'interview schedule' are even more detrimental to developing a satisfactory relationship with the child than they are with the parents. *Flexibility* and *interested listening* are essentials of a good interviewing technique.

Children will often express their feelings in ways other than through words. Here are some examples of drawings produced by children seen in a hospital setting. It is tempting to be over interpretive and read too much into such productions. Nevertheless salient points may often give clues to an examiner as to factors in the child's life which are causing him concern. They may prove a useful starting and talking point for investigations into the child's background.

## References

GRAHAM P. & RUTTER M. (1968). The reliability and validity of the psychiatric assessment of the child. 2. Interview with the parent. *Brit. J. Psychiat.* **114**, 581–592.
RUTTER M., & GRAHAM P. (1968). The reliability and validity of the psychiatric assessment of the child. 1. Interview with the child. *Brit. J. Psychiat.* **114**, 563–579.

## General reading

GOODMAN J.D. & SOURS J.A. (1967). *The Child Mental Status Examination.* New York, Basic Books.
SIMMONS J.E. (1974). *Psychiatric Examination of Children* (2nd ed). Philadelphia, Lea and Febiger.

# Chapter 5

# Psychological Tests

'The time has come' the Walrus said
'To talk of many things:
Of shoes—and ships—and sealing wax—
Of cabbages—and kings—
Any why the sea is boiling hot
And whether pigs have wings.'

Lewis Carroll (Charles Lutwidge Dodgson) 1832–1898
*Through the Looking Glass*

After examining the child the psychiatrist may seek additional information through tests administered and interpreted by a clinical psychologist. Aside from the test results themselves, the psychologist can report on the child's motivation, attention span and general behaviour. Psychological tests serve to confirm a diagnosis or elucidate certain points. They are not themselves, diagnostic. Tests commonly used to assess children can be grouped thus:

● Intelligence tests (tests of cognitive function)
● Educational achievement tests
● Personality assessment (projective) tests
● Tests of motor and perceptual development

Often a 'battery of tests' are administered. Those selected will depend upon where the child's overt problems lie. Needless to say the psychologist requires adequate information on the nature of the problem(s) when the child is referred if the best use is to be made of his/her skills. Most children (and most examiners) enjoy psychological testing.

## INTELLIGENCE TESTS

These are used to assess the child's general ability and to relate this to stadards achieved by others of the same age. The results are summarised as the intelligence quotient—

$$\text{I.Q.} = \frac{\text{Mental Age (as obtained by the test)}}{\text{Chronological Age}} \times 100$$

*Wechsler Intelligence Scale for Children* (W.I.S.C.)

This test is very widely used and regarded as a valuable clinical instrument. It spans the age range 6–15 years and gives a full scale I.Q. which is obtained from two sub-scales as shown in Table 5.1.

| Verbal Scale | Performance Scale |
| --- | --- |
| General information | Picture completion |
| General comprehension | Picture arrangement |
| Arithmetic | Block design |
| Similarities | Object assembly |
| Vocabulary | Coding |
| (Digit span) | (Mazes) |

The last two items in each column are used as alternatives or supplementary tests if time allows. Certain inferences are often drawn from discrepancies between the sub-scales and individual test scores, but there is doubt as to how valid these are. W.I.S.C. intelligence levels are usually grouped as shown in Table 5.2.

| I.Q. | Category |
| --- | --- |
| Below 69 | Mentally subnormal |
| 70– 79 | Borderline mental handicap |
| 80– 89 | Dull normal |
| 90–109 | Normal intelligence |
| 110–119 | Bright normal |
| 120–129 | Superior |
| 130 plus | Very superior |

*Wechsler Pre-school and Primary School Intelligence Scale* (W.P.P.S.I.)

This is a 'downward' extension of the W.I.S.C. designed on the same principles and covers the age range 4–6½ years. It appeals to the interests of young children, is a useful measure of their abilities and very frequently used.

*Stanford Binet Intelligence Scale* (Form L-M)

This is based on the original intelligence test devised by Binet in 1905, but since then has undergone modification and many revisions, the latest by Terman and Merrill in 1960. The tests for younger children involve eye–hand co-ordination, perceptual abilities and naming objects; memory, interpretation of pictures and situations involving practical judgement for older children. There has been some criticism of this test because it is verbally loaded, and individuals with a language handicap or from socially impoverished backgrounds may score relatively poorly. It extends from the age of 2 years to adults, but is generally kept for children.

### *The Coloured Progressive Matrices* (Raven)

This covers the age range 6–13 years. Each test consists of a design or 'matrix' from which a part is missing. The child has to choose from six pieces which is the right one to complete the matrix. This test has the advantage that the material is entirely non-verbal, and can be used by deaf or dysphasic children. It gives a single I.Q. and correlates the W.I.S.C. and Stanford Binet, but cannot be regarded as a substitute for these.

### *McCarthy Scales of Children's Abilities*

This recently introduced test is gaining in popularity, and is appropriate for children from $2\frac{1}{2}$ to $8\frac{1}{2}$ years. Like the W.I.S.C. it has subscales, and these are:

Verbal
Perceptual performance
Quantitative
General cognitive
Memory
Motor

The scale indices give a composite profile of the child's abilities and is particularly useful if he has learning problems at school.

### *The Queensland Test* (D.W. McElwain & G.E. Kearney)

This is a performance test of general cognitive capacity designed for use under conditions of reduced communication. It was developed specifically for selecting persons for training in complex European skills from groups where, because of communication (i.e. language) barriers, the psychological tests usually used for European groups were inapplicable.

### The Goodenough-Harris Drawing Test

This is easily administered and covers children from 5 to 15 years. The child is asked to draw a human figure, or male and female figures, and is scored on the result. The child may produce some interesting asides, for example, the crippled child may reproduce his own handicap as he perceives it.

### Tests for younger children

In general these are not as reliable as tests for older children, but the skill and experience of the psychologist will influence the value of the results. *The Merrill-Palmer* scale covers the ages 18 months to 6 years, and consists of verbal and non-verbal items. The result is usually expressed as a mental age and gives a useful general estimate of the child's abilities. *The Griffiths Mental Developmental Scale* covers the first two years of life. There are five sections, locomotor, personal–social, hearing and speech, eye and hand, and performance, from these a mental age is derived. *The Gesell developmental schedule* covers the age range 4 weeks to 6 years and has four sections—motor, language, adaptive behaviour, and personal–social. It is scored as a developmental age, and from this the developmental quotient (D.Q.) is obtained.

$$D.Q. = \frac{\text{Developmental age}}{\text{Chronological age}} \times 100$$

*The Cattell Scale* is a 'downward' extension of the Stanford Binet and covers the ages 2 to 30 months. *The Bayley Scale of Mental and Motor Development* takes items from tests described above (those which by standardisation, have proved to be the most useful), and adds new ones. It is considered the best standardised infant scale today. Developmental screening tests for infants in paediatric clinics, for example, that devised by Sheridan, are not administered by psychologists nor standardised in the same way as are the tests described here (see p. 36).

### The value of intelligence tests

Psychological tests must be valid (i.e. measure what they set out to measure) and reliable (i.e. give consistent scores for the same individual when they are repeated). On the whole, tests for older children are more reliable. Validity raises the question of what we are trying to measure in an intelligence test. A discussion of this is outside the scope of this book, but the practical value of these tests lies in the correlation between results and abilities required for learning and success at school. This does not say that the child will succeed, but that he has the potential to do so. He may achieve poorly because of emotional and personality factors; assessment of these will be described in the next section.

There has been some criticism that giving a child an intelligence quotient may saddle him with a label which sticks for a very long time, although in fact the only inference which should be drawn from the result is that he was functioning at a specific level at the time he did the test. There is now a tendency to describe the child as functioning within a certain 'band' or range, and for the psychologist to qualify this by reporting factors which might have influenced his performance.

## TESTS OF EDUCATIONAL ACHIEVEMENT

These give a profile of how the child actually performs at school in different subjects, and when judged in relation to his general intelligence may reveal areas of particular difficulty. Generally they should be supplemented by a teacher's report. The commonly used ones in Australian schools are as follows:

### Schonell Attainment and Diagnostic Tests of Reading

There are four sub-tests. R1 is a graded word recognition test; 100 words are arranged in a progressive order of difficulty and the test covers the range 5 to 15 years, 10 words per year are given which a child of a specific age should be able to read. R2, R3 and R4 are tests of reading comprehension which cover successively more difficult levels from age 6 to 13 years. In R2 a passage is read aloud and scored for speed, accuracy and comprehension. R3 and R4 are silent reading tests followed by questions, and test memory as well as comprehension and reading ability.

### The Standard Reading Tests (Daniels and Diak)

These consist of a battery of 12 tests which assess different aspects of reading skills. A six monthly assessment on test 1 is recommended, and if performance causes concern, a more detailed diagnosis of the situation can be undertaken by using tests 2–12.

### Schonell Diagnostic English Tests

These cover the use of English generally, capital letters, punctuation and so on. A profile of attainment in English is derived for the child.

### Neale Analysis of Reading Ability

This covers the 6 to 13 years range and qualitative information is gained regarding general reading habits and word recognition.

### Schonell Arithmetic Attainment and Diagnostic Tests

These are available in mechanical and problem arithmetic for children between 7 and 15 years. They give a picture of attainment in various areas of arithmetic and allow weakness to be investigated. Unfortunately these tests are of less value because rapidly changing methods of teaching mathematics have tended to make them unreliable.

### Wide Range Achievement Test (W.R.A.T.)

This gives an overall picture of the child's school achievement in reading, spelling and arithmetic.

## PERSONALITY ASSESSMENT

An attempt is made to gain an understanding of the child as a whole by assessing personality traits and attitudes. Three general methods are used:

### 1. Projective techniques

The child is presented with ambiguous (usually visual) stimuli, for example a vague shape or picture, and asked to interpret what he sees. In so doing he projects upon it his way of perceiving life, i.e. the examiner sees into the child's world. There are several of these tests and although the interpretation of them is difficult, they can be of value in the clinical situation. For example:

The child is shown a picture of a car about to go over a cliff and is asked how he feels about it. The aggressive child says: 'Let them go, it will be a good smash'; the conscientious and responsible child devises means of stopping it; and the nervous child suggests methods of keeping out of the way in case he is hurt himself.

*The Rorschach Test* using inkblots is widely known, but the *Children's Apperception Test* (C.A.T.) is more commonly used. The child is presented with pictures about which he must tell a story. The *Bene-Anthony Family Relations Test* taps information about emotional relationships within the family. It consists of a series of figures representing members of the family, plus one figure labelled 'nobody'. Each figure has a box attached, the child is given cards on which statements are written, for example 'This person is the strongest', and is asked to 'post' them into the most appropriate box.

These tests do not have the scientific approach of intellectual or educational tests, nevertheless they may supplement information derived from the child's clinical interview. Asking for *drawings of family and home*, *telling a story* about another child, or asking for *three favourite wishes* are all methods of projective assessment and are commonly used in psychiatric interviews.

## 2. Psychometrics

The *Junior Eysenck Personality Inventory* for 7 to 16-year-olds, and the *Children's Personality Questionnaire* (C.P.Q.) for 6 to 16 years devised by Cattell, attempt to measure personality attributes by assessing the child's replies to a series of questions. Both have built-in 'lie' scores and have been standardised on large numbers of children. They represent an advance on projective tests in the scientific study of personality.

## 3. The Bristol Social Adjustment Guides

The Bristol Social Adjustment Guides are also based on questionnaires, and different versions are used in relation to the child at school, the child in residential care, the child in the family, and for boys and girls. They offer a method of detecting and diagnosing maladjustment and tension in school-age children, but their predictive value is unknown.

## TESTS OF MOTOR AND PERCEPTUAL DEVELOPMENT

These are valuable for children with learning problems and where neurological deficits are suspected.

### *Lincoln-Oseretsky Motor Development Scale*

This test efficiently measures motor skills (both fine and gross movements), and allows comparison with children of the same age. A motor development quotient can be calculated and compared with the individual's intellectual level, scholastic achievement and social skills. It is of particular value in assessing children referred because of clumsiness, and whose motor dysfunction may have an important bearing on education and vocation.

### *Bender Visual-Motor Gestalt Test*

In this test the child copies a series of figures and it is claimed that the score he obtains may help to establish a diagnosis of brain damage. It is widely used and taps certain aspects of visual-motor performance in children from 4 to 12 years, but to what extent it assesses brain damage *per se* is uncertain.

### *Beery-Buktenica Test of Visual-Motor Integration*

This also taps visual-perceptual and visual-motor skills, and gives a visual perceptual age level.

### *Frostig Test of Visual Perception* and *Wepman Auditory Discrimination Test*

Assess visual and auditory perceptual skills respectively.

## Summary

In this overview of commonly used psychological tests, emphasis has been given to those administered on an individual basis, for this usually obtains in clinic practice. Some, particularly educational tests, can be given to groups of children, but they are less reliable and the child who is not co-operating well, for example because of emotional disturbance, illness or tiredness, may be wrongly judged.

## CLINICAL EXAMPLES

*Simon*, aged 10.8 years, was referred with the following comments:
● He is bottom of his class and parents call him stupid, slow and clumsy.
● He enjoys social activities but seems quite unable to catch a ball. Children tease him and refuse to play with him.
● He is called 'isolated', 'withdrawn' and 'weary looking' by his teacher.

History and clinical examination showed minor neurological handicaps (minimal brain dysfunction), motor co-ordination was particularly poor.

The psychologists report was as follows:
'Simon was not well motivated to achieve in the test situation. He either complained that tasks presented to him were too difficult or attempted to distract the examiner. His results on the *Wechsler Intelligence Scale for Children* were:

| | |
|---|---|
| Verbal Score | I.Q. 106 |
| Performance Score | I.Q. 92 |
| Full Scale Score | I.Q. 100' |

The difference of 14 points between the verbal and performance scores is statistically significant and indicative of perceptual problems. These are also suggested by his very low scores on block design (reproducing patterns using coloured blocks) and coding.

*The Beery Buktenica Test of Visual-Motor Integration* gives an age equivalent of 7.10 years.

Although of normal intelligence, this boy is hampered in his school work by perceptual difficulties and poor motor coordination. In tasks involving eye-hand coordination such as writing or copying figures from the blackboard, he functions at a level nearly 3 years below his chronological age.

*Tina* was 11 years old when she was seen; her parents complained of her inability to follow instructions, periods of daydreaming, difficulties with school work especially reading. Her assessment was as follows:
*Wechsler Intelligence Scale for Children*

|               |          |      |
|---------------|----------|------|
| Verbal Score  | I.Q.     | 80   |
| Performance Score | I.Q. | 100  |
| Full Scale Score | I.Q.  | 92   |

*Neal Analysis of Reading Ability* showed a reading age of 8.9 years, i.e. 2.3 years behind her chronological age.

During the session the psychologist noted that Tina was often slow to comprehend instructions and seemed very anxious. She would divert the conversation if subjects were introduced which involved the use of complicated words and mispronounced many words, e.g. piropacter for chiropractor (her father's occupation). Tina's hearing was perfect but she suffered from a specific language disability (congenital dysphasia). Language development had been slow, she only produced simple sentences by 3 years of age. Although potentially of average intelligence, she was frustrated by her handicap and the situation was made worse by her parents complaints of laziness and unfavourable comparisons with her sisters. Her school work had been hampered throughout by her failure to comprehend spoken and written instructions. Understandably she became anxious when asked to display her language ability, and would 'cut off' into daydreams.

*Jane* was 3.7 years old when she was referred because of her negativistic behaviour in kindergarten. She was the only child of indulgent elderly parents who thought she could do no wrong. Her kindergarten teacher, who knew the family well, referred to her as 'spoilt', 'self-centred' and 'demanding'. The report on her psychological assessment was as follows: 'Jane approached the test situation rather hesitantly, she seemed eager to be involved, but showed a high level of anxiety when presented with tasks. Her attention span was good and she related warmly to the examiner.

Her profile on the *McCarthy Scale of Children's Abilities* was as follows:

|                           |           |
|---------------------------|-----------|
| Verbal scale              | +2  S.D.  |
| Perceptual performance scale | +1  S.D. |
| Quantitative scale        | +1.5 S.D. |
| General cognitive scale   | +1.5 S.D. |
| Memory scale              | +2  S.D.  |
| Motor scale               | −2.5 S.D. |

Jane's estimated mental age is 4.9 years (intelligence quotient 126). Her good verbal ability reflects her background, where she is constantly in the company of adults. Her motor deficit is, however, a considerable handicap to her. She was noted to be clumsy in her movements and it is not surprising her parents call her 'accident prone'. One wonders to what extent their overprotection has hampered her in the development of fine motor skills. She had certainly become anxious about performing motor tasks. Her teacher's criticism probably aggravates her kindergarten behaviour.'

*General Reading*

SAVAGE R.D. 1968. *Psychometric Assessment of the Individual Child.* Ringwood, Victoria. Penguin Books, Australia Ltd.

# Chapter 6
# The Child in Today's Society


## ENVIRONMENTAL FACTORS WHICH MAY
## AFFECT A CHILD'S ADJUSTMENT


'Circumstances alter cases'

Charles Dickens (1812–1870)
*Edwin Drood. Chapter 9.*


Factors associated with psychiatric disturbance in childhood were discussed in Chapter 3. This chapter describes life situations which are potentially damaging to children. Chapters 7 and 8 look at reactions shown by children, to stress.

The emotional climate of the home has profound significance for personality development in the early years. To be without dependable parent figures is one of the greatest misfortunes life has to offer. Loss of parents or deficiencies in the quality of parenting a child receives, may lead to serious disturbance in childhood or later life. Consideration is therefore first given to situations where parents are unable to fill their role adequately, then to the absence of parents and ways and means of providing parent substitutes. Social and cultural factors impinging upon children today will also be discussed.

Inadequate parental care may result in timid and anxious or rebellious and antisocial children. However, some cope surprisingly well, even developing a protective attitude toward disturbed parents. The presence of others in the environment, e.g. older siblings or grandparents, who can respond to the child's needs can mitigate the effects of deficient parenting.


## PARENTAL DISTURBANCE

Rutter (1966) studied the effects of sick and disturbed parents upon children. His conclusions were:
● The younger the child the greater is the likelihood of reactive disturbance.

● Temperamental differences are obviously important; a placid child may cope with family stress better than a tense one.

● Boys are more susceptible to environmental disturbance than girls.

● The effect of parental illness may be related more to the disruption of family life and social difficulties it entails, rather than to clinical symptoms shown by the parent. This is particularly true of psychosis unless the child becomes involved in a parent's delusional system and his perception by the parent is seriously distorted.

● Parents with long standing abnormalities of personality are more likely to produce behavioural disturbances in their children than those with severe, but shortlived illness.

● Although neurosis in parents has a less flamboyant symptomatology than psychosis, it may have more serious effects upon the child's personality development.

Modern management of adult psychiatric patients tends toward keeping them in the community and living at home as much as possible. Although commendable from their point of view, the effect it has upon their families, especially young children, should be considered and this is by no means always the case.

*Immature and inadequate parents* find child rearing a difficult task and often become unduly dependent upon clinics and welfare agencies seeking supportive figures (virtually parents for themselves) who can care for them when the family situation becomes more than they can manage. Many such personalities marry in an effort to satisfy dependency needs, i.e. look for a relationship which gives care and protection but to which they contribute nothing in return, and often find a partner with the same problem. When this manœuvre fails, as it is almost certain to do, they turn to their offspring for support. Since the young child is incapable of giving this the parent becomes angry, sometimes with disastrous results (see violence to children). The role of the family doctor in giving supportive care to these families is important, especially if he is at hand in times of crisis. Support can be given in a general practice setting, but it calls for a nice balance between meeting the parent's dependency needs and encouraging their independence. *Neurotic families* is the term used by Wolff (1973) to describe homes in which unresolved childhood conflicts of parents continually interfere with the way in which the children are managed. Although superficially these families appear stable, united and respectable, home life is characterised by frustration and discontent. Sometimes in an effort to solve his own difficulties, a parent may covertly encourage one type of behaviour in his child while overtly condemning it, trapping the child in a double-bind; whatever he does is wrong. Understandably, such management may be associated with serious personality distortion in the child. *Sociopathic behaviour* in parents is understandably reflected in children. Parental example seems more likely to produce delinquency in the offspring than any supposed genetic influences. *Alcoholism in parents* may result in much abuse and neglect of children. Crisis centres which offer protection from a drunken and abusive father are being established in large cities and more are needed. Societies such as Alanon have developed in an effort to give help and social support to the relatives of people who drink to excess.

Anthony (1969) studied the children of *psychotic (schizophrenic) parents*. He reported that many learned to adapt to a double standard of reality, accepting both the irrational orientation at home and the differing standards at school. Some children attempted to cover for their parent's irrational behaviour, others accepted their parent's delusions, while a few, particularly younger ones, showed behaviour which Anthony believed might be a precursor of psychotic illness in later life.

## CHILDREN'S PHYSICAL COMPLAINTS AS A SIGN OF PARENTAL DISTURBANCE

It is fairly obvious that behavioural disturbance in a child may be indicative of family pathology, however the situation may not be so easily recognised when physical complaints in children are involved. Anxiety, depression or hypochondriasis in a mother may result in repeated requests to treat a midly infected throat or a barely perceptable cough. Depression is commonly encountered in general practice. It is estimated that per 1,000 head of population, each practitioner has an annual case load of 14 to 22 patients suffering from depression (Watts 1966). Although these will usually present with typical symptoms, a child's physical complaints, behavioural disturbance or even perceived disturbance may be the presenting symptom of a psychiatrically ill, often depressed parent. The commonest reason for failing to recognise depression is failing to consider the possibility of such a diagnosis. Every patient who is significantly depressed is at risk of suicide, and when it is a parent of young children, other lives can be at risk as well.

## VIOLENCE TO CHILDREN – PSYCHIATRIC ASPECTS

The term 'Battered Child Syndrome' has come into general use to describe children suffering from non-accidental injury by a caretaker, usually a parent.


## Prevalence

We do not know whether today's children suffer from this type of violence more frequently than children did in the past. It is possible that modern conditions such as small families, compact houses and flats and social mobility (which separates young parents from the support of older relatives) contribute toward increased tension between family members and this erupts in violence. Since Kempe first drew attention to the seriousness of the problem (Kempe *et al.* 1962), there has been an increasing awareness that children damaged physically by parents are not uncommon. The real prevalence rate is not known, but it is generally agreed that recognised cases are only the 'tip of the iceberg'. Large numbers of children suffering from injury and from physical and psychological neglect go unrecorded. The injury may be concealed by parents and even today professional staff may be ignorant or reluctant to report cases as they fear litigation.

In Britain it is estimated that as many as 700 children a year die as the result of violence (Renvoize 1975). Birrell and Birrell (1968) reported the detection of over one case a month at the Royal Children's Hospital, Melbourne, which serves a population of two and a half million. Kempe estimates that the syndrome occurs as commonly as 6/1,000 live births, and that the mortality rate among abused children is at least 10% (Scott 1977).


## The children

Those damaged are young, generally under 4 years and often under one. They may be singletons or members of small families and are more often boys than girls. There is often some factor present likely to affect the early mother–child relationship, such as illegitimacy or prematurity or the child suffers from a physical or mental handicap. The children are often dirty, unkempt and malnourished; 'failure to thrive' is a common presenting symptom, but this is not always so; they may appear to be well cared for. Older children can be emotionally frozen, they cower in a corner crying silently, since they have learned that to make a noise brings retribution. The psychological damage which accompanies violence may be even worse in the long run than the physical injury incurred.

## The parents

Parents who maltreat their children are also young, say between 18 and 25 years. They are not always in poor socio-economic conditions, but many are. They seldom suffer from psychiatric illness *per se*, but from long standing personality difficulties with persistent emotional problems and feelings of frustration relating to their own childhood experiences, which are often of deprivation and cruelty. In this respect, one generation tends to hand on to the next patterns of bad parenting involving physical violence. One study (Oliver 1971) has revealed five generations of child abuse.

There are often indications that the family has been in precarious adjustment for some time, often because of material worries, such as unemployment, bad debts or poor housing. Alcoholism may be a contributory factor. A comparatively trivial incident or a child's incessant whining triggers a sudden loss of control and an aggressive attack is made on the defenceless child. Sometimes 'punishment' gets out of hand. Three types of parental personality appear to be involved:

1 The habitually aggressive who vent their feelings on the nearest source of irritation, e.g. the crying child. These people are unstable and may be mentally dull. Smith (Smith *et al.* 1973) suggests that aggressive psychopaths, a number of whom have abnormal electroencephalograms may form a proportion of this group.

2 Immature personalities who cannot sustain a child-nurturing relationship and expect the child to meet their needs, rather than the reverse.

3 The third group are an extension of the second in that they are basically emotionally impoverished but they cope with their difficulties by adopting rigid and controlling attitudes, and are unable to tolerate normal childish, 'disobedient' behaviour. Some perceive the child as their own bad childhood self, and any minor misdeed on the child's part is 'punished' to excess.

More females than males damage children; perhaps this is because the child spends a greater proportion of his time in the mother's company. Dalton (1975) has reported that violence to children occurs commonly during the mother's premenstruum when she is tired and irritable. Although one parent is usually responsible for the damage, the other often colludes or may encourage the battering, for example, by suggesting the child is spoiled and needs punishment.

## Psychiatric sequelae in the child

Brain injury resulting in mental subnormality is not uncommon since children are often beaten about the head. Distorted attitudes toward parent figures and maladjustment have been described. Perhaps the most tragic outcome of all is that these children never learn what good parenting means and may become emotionally depriving and violent parents in their turn.

## Presentation of battered children

This is dealt with in paediatric texts; briefly typical features are:
● Repeated visits to hospital or surgery with minor injuries ('the cry for help'). Follow-up appointments are not kept.
● A delay between the 'accident' and the presentation for advice or parents may rush to a casualty department at an unlikely hour, sometimes showing anxiety out of proportion to the degree of damage.
● Lesions are dispersed in time and site, thus bruises are in various sites and of different ages.
● Epiphyseal detachment, spiral fractures of the long bones, and dislocated elbows and shoulders are common. The injuries are unlikely to have been incurred by a young child; fractures in a non-walking child should arouse suspicion. Cigarette burns on arms or back and human bite marks are not uncommon.
● Malnutrition and neglect.

## Management

Obviously the child must be removed from the parents' care, at least as a temporary measure, and in general practice or casualty work, immediate admission to hospital is the best way of ensuring this. Subsequently the State child welfare department must be involved. Many parents are acutely distressed by what has happened and given adequate time with a sympathetic listener, are willing to discuss their need for help. They must not be antagonised by accusations which could be ill founded.

There has been much discussion as to whether child abuse should be made a compulsorily notifiable condition, and recently legislation has been introduced to ensure this in two States. Notification does not mean that parents will be punished. In general a punitive approach has not been found helpful.

## Can child abuse be prevented?

Continuing education relating to child abuse for those in contact with young children is very important. The public need reassurance that they can give information to welfare agencies in confidence and that they will not be blamed for 'telling tales'. It is important to get across to families that hospitals and other agencies exist to help and not to punish.

Kempe and his team (Kempe 1973) in Denver recognise that many women are unable to give good quality mothering for twenty-four hours a day, 7 days a week, and the provision of substitute child care for short periods in families where a mother is under considerable stress or has shown herself to have limited patience with young children could prevent the build up of tension which results in child abuse. It is claimed that information obtained during the pregnancy, and observation of the mother's reaction to her baby at birth may indicate the potential to abuse (Lynch *et al.* 1976).

## Should battered children be returned to their parents?

The aim should be to settle abused children back with their families eventually. Many parents will need support and help in practical ways, e.g. with housing or finance. Contraceptive advice is necessary since another child would represent a further risk.

Kempe employs social workers to supervise untrained 'mothering aides' who help the families. These women, selected on their ability to be flexible, non-critical and non-directive, establish close contact with a family who has abused a child. The family is able to telephone their aide (or a well-known substitute) at any hour of the day or night if tension rises and they fear losing control. Kempe's team claims to have returned children safely to their families within eight months of an incident of battering, and in several hundred families no further abuse has occurred. If such a service cannot be arranged, the provision of a twenty-four hours telephone service or crisis centre offers an alternative.

## THE SPECTRUM OF CHILD ABUSE

Aside from physical violence and the emotional trauma which accompanies it, the maltreatment syndrome has been broadened to encompass nutritional, medical care and safety neglect as well as drug and sexual abuse (Schmitt & Kempe 1975). The administration of non-prescribed drugs to young children has been reported by Rogers *et al.* (1976) and sexual misuse (defined as exposure to sexual stimulation inappropriate to age, level of psychosexual development and role in the family) by Brant and Tisza (1977). Incestuous relationships, between fathers and their daughters are probably more common than is generally recognised and associated often with total family dysfunction, the mothers being aware of the relationship but choosing to deny it or to collude with their husbands (*Brit. Med. J.* 1972). Although it is hard to separate the effects of the incestuous relationship from those of other pathology in the background, Lukianowicz (1972) describes psychopathy, promiscuity, frigidity after marriage and psychiatric disturbance (neurotic symptoms) as sequelae among the girls.

Child murder by parents may be the end result of the abuse syndrome. However, other dynamics are often involved (Resnick 1969). Thus a depressed parent who sees no hope for the future may kill both himself and his child, especially if the latter suffers from mental or physical handicap. Occasionally an illegitimate child is destroyed, often at birth; rarely a psychotic parent may attack a child in response to hallucinatory voices or because he holds some delusion about his being evil.

## ILLEGITIMATE CHILDREN

Children of single mothers are from the start at a disadvantage and at risk of developing physical and emotional handicaps (*Lancet* 1972). Perinatal morbidity rates are high and social and material difficulties likely later on. Children who remain with their mothers show a higher incidence of behavioural and school problems than those placed in adoptive homes soon after birth. Since the conception of an illegitimate child may represent one stage in a life of repeated social failures, the mother may be handicapped by her own personality before she attempts childrearing. Of course there are well-adjusted individuals who cope successfully; there is less stigma attached to illegitimacy nowadays and monetary support is easier, but the mother needs to be made aware of the stresses inherent in the situation. She must decide for herself whether or not to keep her child without pressure from parents or well meaning relatives. otherwise she may be left with long lasting feelings of remorse and guilt. She should be made aware it is often hard to find an adoptive home for an older child should she wish to relinquish him later. Teenage pregnancies are discussed on p. 212.

## PARENTAL DIVORCE

Loss of a parent through separation or divorce is a relatively common experience in childhood today; it is estimated that one in four marriages break irretrievably before the children of the marriage reach school leaving age (*Brit. Med. J.* 1972). Parental divorce inevitably leaves its mark upon children; the following effects have been described:

● Divorce represents bereavement for many children with the same fear, guilt – the child feels responsible for the break-up of the marriage – and need to mourn the lost parent.

● Disturbed behaviour often antisocial, in character (Brown 1968) and depression (McDermott 1970) are common. Boys appear to be most vulnerable to parental divorce.

● Divorce is a *process*, and the constant quarrelling and divided loyalties experienced beforehand may produce this disturbed behaviour, rather than the separation itself. In some instances the child may benefit from the relief of tension once the divorce is through.

● Divorce is often accompanied by a drop in the standard of living; this, together with the lack of discipline which often obtains in a one parent family, may be the reason for lower educational achievement in these children when compared with children whose families are intact.

The Family Law Act (1975) makes the welfare of the child a paramount consideration in divorce cases, allows his wishes to be taken into account and for him to be represented by counsel when decisions regarding his custody are made. Although laudable, this may result in parents battling to gain favour with their child and raises questions as to what the child's primary needs are and who briefs his advocate. Goldstein *et al.* (1973) draw attention to the young child's need for continuous relationships with adults, to his inability to cope with delays while decisions as to placement are being made and the law's incapacity to supervise interpersonal relationships on a long term basis. Undoubtedly a panel of individuals who know the child well is the best approach to determining satisfactory custody arrangements but no court can compensate a child for the loss of a parent.

# BEREAVEMENT IN CHILDHOOD

The concept of death may be slow to develop in modern childhood; contact with death, e.g. through the loss of a sibling, is infrequent. Less attention is paid to religious beliefs and in many families, 'death has replaced sex as the great taboo'. Books have therefore been prepared to help parents introduce the subject to children and some are listed at the end of this chapter. There are differences between losing a parent through death and through divorce. Society is more supportive of the bereaved family and generally the parental quarrels which precede the loss of a parent through divorce and which are so detrimental to the child are absent. Following the death of a parent one has to consider:

## Immediate reactions

● These depend to some extent upon the age and temperament of the child and the ability of the surviving parent to fill two roles. The finality of death cannot be fully appreciated until the age of 8 or 9 years.
● Young children may show little overt grief and this apparent may be regarded as callous, however it relates to bewilderment and fear lest the other parent 'disappears' as well.
● Older children may worry about what has happened to the body, about ghosts and the material circumstances of the family.
● The child may feel deserted and angry and he may direct hostility toward the surviving parent for allowing the other to go.
● Sometimes the child may blame himself for the death (see p. 143 reactions of siblings).
● During the process of mourning many people become cut off and isolated from others. When this happens to the surviving parent it virtually has the effect of depriving the child of both parents for a while.

## Long term effects

● There is evidence that death of a parent may be an aetiological factor in delinquent behaviour in childhood and psychiatric disturbance in later life. Brown (1961) and Greer (1964) have shown there is a higher incidence of depression and of suicide in adults who lose parents in childhood. It has been suggested that the individual becomes sensitised to loss through this event, and overreacts to real or perceived loss subsequently, rather in the manner of an amaphylactic reaction. Social problems resultant to the loss of a breadwinner and lack of discipline and an identificatory figure are all important (Rutter 1966).

### Advising the bereaved family

A period of mourning to work through feelings in relation to the deceased and come to terms with the fact there will be no return, is as necessary for children as everyone else. It is helpful if the older child can discuss the death with a responsible adult whose ideas relating to death are congruent with those of the family. Bonds are strengthened if the family members remain together during the period of adjustment, unless the surviving parent is seriously disturbed. Older children should not be excluded from the events associated with the death, for example, kept away from a parent's funeral. It is better to know what happens to the deceased than to imagine what could have occurred. Witnessing adults' public expressions of grief may help a child to express his own. Many older children will show a remarkably mature response to the family situation, acting as substitute parents for younger siblings and helping with the practical aspects of family life.

## CHILDREN 'IN CARE'

In the event of a child losing both parents and if his family are unable to provide for him, he becomes the responsibility of the State Children's Welfare Department. Recognition of the detrimental effects upon children of impersonal management in institutions has resulted in efforts to find substitute parents for them whenever possible. Large orphanages have been replaced by 'cottage homes'. Here small groups of children, preferably of different ages, as would obtain in a family, live with a husband and wife couple (who are employed to care for them) in a house which differs very little from others in the same street and suburb. Other arrangements are also described.

# ADOPTION

This has become an increasingly popular means of providing substitute care for children when parents die, or for one reason or another, relinquish all their rights to the child. Between eighty and ninety percent of adopted children are illegitimate (Seglow *et al.* 1972). Most adoptions work well, but certain considerations are necessary to ensure success:

## *The age of the child at adoption*

Whenever possible the arrangements should be made in the early weeks of life; after the child has reached 2 years, adoption is less likely to be successful.

## *Parents attitudes*

Adopting a child is a most rewarding experience but is not identical with biological parenthood. Parents may be disappointed if this is not explained to them. An adopted child cannot replace a lost natural child (he's a unique individual) nor cement a shaky marriage. If he serves as a continual reminder of his adoptive parents infertility or is taken expressly on the wishes of one partner and reluctantly by the other, difficulties may occur. Children do not show gratitude, at least in the early years and those who take them must not expect or demand it. Most children at times conjure up fantasy parents – generally without the shortcomings they perceive in their own – adoptive parents must be reassured that this is a normal phase and does not indicate a lack of affection on the child's part.

## *Matching children and parents*

Where the child's physical and intellectual attributes fit in well with those of his adoptive family, this is ideal. Adoption agencies do their best to place children appropriately but because of the age at which children go to adoptive families, this is by no means easy. The natural parents socioeconomic status has proved a useful predictor of their child's intellectual level. If physical or intellectual handicap develops, many adoptive parents find it harder to accept than if the child were their own. Careful physical examination of the child is essential prior to arranging adoption. There are families who are well able to make a home for a handicapped child, but in such a case the parents should be informed of all the known facts before they undertake his care. (*Brit. Med. J.* 1977) Particular difficulties arise if a natural parent is known to suffer from mental handicap or illness e.g. schizophrenia.

### Preparation for adoption

It is obvious that a couple's motives for wishing to adopt must be assessed prior to placement of a young baby with them. A social worker's assistance is valuable both from this point of view and for answering questions which may arise subsequently.

### When should we tell the child of his adoption?

All prospective adoptive parents ask this. Where it is not done, sooner or later it is discovered by the child and may have unhappy consequences. It is wisest to bring the child up telling him he is adopted and gradually explain the meaning of this to him.

### Emotional disturbance in adopted children

Child Guidance Clinic figures show a greater than expected proportion of adopted children among their clients; 5–13% of their referrals relate to adopted children, compared with the prevalence of adoption of 2% in the population at large (Wolff 1973). This may reflect the adoptive parents' zeal to be good parents and familiarity with social agencies to some extent, but the prevalence of behaviour disorders does appear to be higher in adopted children. This may be associated with several factors, described under 'illegitimate children' (p. 80).

## FOSTER CARE

When the child is likely to return to his natural parents after some time, especially if he is very young, fostering offers an opportunity for life within a family. If concern is felt about a child being handicapped and a period of observation prior to arranging his adoption is necessary, this arrangement is also valuable. The child remains the responsibility of his legal guardian (usually the State) and is placed in the home of a married couple who are paid for his maintenance. It is true that the emotional relationships developed with the foster family will have to be broken, but this is better than institutional life for the child.

## STEP-PARENTS

Reactions to an outsider entering the family in the role of a parent are variable depending upon the age and sex of the child, the sex of the step-parent and the circumstances under which the event occurs. However, loyalty to a parent remains even if the child has been treated harshly and the substitute parent may be rejected as a usurper or at the best treated ambivalently. It may require much tact and patience on his part to resolve this conflict of loyalties. Where the step-parent brings children of his own, efforts must be directed toward the 'mixed' family developing an identity of its own.

## SOCIO-CULTURAL DEPRIVATION, MULTI-PROBLEM FAMILIES

The socially disadvantaged child is defined as one who lacks the opportunities for healthy growth and development which are available to the majority of his peers. He comes (generally) from the slums of large industrial towns and suffers from both physical and pscyhological environmental deficiencies (*Brit. Med. J.* 1976).

● His pregnancy is likely to be poorly supervised and the mother's nutrition inadequate.

● During childhood, deficiencies in diet and hygiene render him liable to frequent infections which are often inadequately treated. He may be apathetic, anaemic or subject to chronic disease; commonly ears and upper respiratory tract are affected. He is liable to periods of deafness when he is called stupid and shouted at.

● At home, language development is not encouraged. In his background, body language, grimaces and monosyllabic utterances (mostly shouts) are the currency of communication. He does not develop the ability to express his feeling in words, but when tension rises learns to erupt into aggressive behaviour.

● His background is unstimulating, no one reads to him, he does not have the opportunity to practice skills likely to be of use later at school, such as how to manipulate pencils, scissors or paints.

● Discipline is inconsistent. No one reasons with him. He is coerced into obedience generally by physical methods.

● Mother interprets exploratory behaviour as aggressive and punishes it, and he comes to lack initiative.

● He adopts parental attitudes of mistrust toward authority figures, e.g. father evades the police so he avoids contact with the child welfare workers.

● He does not learn to plan for the future, because the family live from hand to mouth. He is impulsive and grabs what he can in his precarious existence.

Needless to say he measures up poorly when he starts school with its middle class ethos. He relates badly to the teacher, lacks motivation (father persistently points out to him the futility of learning – he found no use for it himself) and fine motor and language skills. His attendance record is poor often because he is kept home to mind siblings. All in all, he starts school likely to fail, and drop out, and there is a considerable chance that he will become delinquent. If he is picked up by the police for some transgression, it is likely that he will be brought before the court as other members of his family are known to be 'troublesome', whereas a child from a different background would only be cautioned.

In spite of all this, he is precocious in survival techniques in his specific environment. He is skilled in caring for himself and his siblings, in doing housework, and dealing with drunken parents. Gross motor development is advanced, he has had to fend for himself from early life. Such skills are not capitalised in our educational system.

### Social versus emotional deprivation

Although many of the children described above come from unstable and emotionally depriving backgrounds, for example, the father is absent for gaol sentences or mother deserts her family from time to time, this is by no means always the case. There may be emotional warmth and intense loyalty in such families. *Social and emotional deprivation are not synonomous.* An overzealous welfare agency that removes a child from a socially depriving background may be removing him from emotional support as well. Both facets of deprivation must be carefully appraised before action is taken.

*Cycles of deprivation; prevention of sociocultural deprivation*

Life styles are perpetuated from one generation to the next. Preventive measures must attempt to break this vicious circle. Programmes, such as operation headstart in the U.S.A., have been directed towards improving nutrition, hygiene and environmental stimulation from infancy to the start of school, utilising a day kindergarten setting. These have not been an unqualified success, but much has been learned from them. The children involved cope better at the start of school, but unless the extra help is continued into school years, their performance starts to fall as their environment cannot sustain the improvement. Working with the families as well as with the children improves the situation, and also prevents alienation of the child from his background, which may occur if behaviour and attitudes in the child are changed without a change occurring in the parents' orientation.


# ETHNIC AND CULTURAL DIFFERENCES. MINORITY GROUPS

## Aboriginal children

What has been said in the preceding section is often applicable to Aboriginal children living under urban conditions in Australia. They are labelled dull because of their failure to progress in the classroom. Standard intelligence tests tend to underestimate these children since they are loaded in favour of verbal ability and Western society norms. An intelligence test has been devised for Aboriginals (Queensland Test, see p. 64) which avoids these factors and gives an opportunity for accurate assessment.

Identity problems may be considerable, especially around adolescence. A 12-years-old part-Aboriginal boy presented with symptoms of anxiety and depression expressed by stealing and senseless acts of vandalism. He was called 'blacky' at school where he was the only Aboriginal boy in his class, and 'whitey' at home where his skin was lighter than most of the extended family with whom he lived. He lacked a sense of belonging, was bewildered and angry. Casework enabled him to adjust to his difficulties to some extent, but his problem is a major one for Aboriginal youth in Australian society today.

### Children of migrants

Children pick up the language and culture of Australian society quickly and often settle more rapidly than their parents. There may be clashes because standards imposed at home differ from those at school. This is likely to be accentuated where the parents spend much of their time with other migrants of similar background to their own. Social worker involvement with the families in an attempt to resolve differences and efforts to help the parents integrate better into Australian society, e.g. attendance at language classes, may help toward a solution.

## MATERNAL EMPLOYMENT OUTSIDE THE HOME

### The rights and wrongs

Research into this area is difficult because of the number of variables involved. The age of the child, the mother's attitude to work, her adequacy in filling two roles and the quality of substitute care she provides are factors to be considered in assessing the effects on the child. There is no doubt that pre-school children 'dumped' in overcrowded nurseries, where they receive scant attention from adults, suffer physically and psychologically, especially as the mother may be too tired to do much for the child in the hours she does spend with him. 'Latch key' children who come home from school before mother returns from work are a current social problem. Sometimes they remain locked out (one mother told the writer she feared her son would break the television set) and wander the streets unsupervised and hungry. It is not surprising they get into trouble.

Older children, whose mothers find job satisfaction and provide adequate supervision in their absence, have been shown to benefit from their mother working, and show advanced verbal and social skills (Wallston 1973). A satisfied working mother may be a better companion to her family than an unsatisfied, non-working one. However, there is much confusion in the public mind and maternal employment is broadly and often unjustifiably equated with maternal deprivation. This results in a feeling of guilt in those who have to work from sheer necessity. Others, inspired by groups in society who denigrate the value of homemaking and rearing children, feel guilty because they don't. Between these extremes are many variations, and when assessing effects on children, each family must be judged individually.

*Summary and recommendations*

● Society must accept that mothers employed outside the home are a feature of modern life and an important work force.

● Public money is needed to provide adequate substitute care in créches for young children and for supervised playgrounds for children unable to return home directly after school.

● If a woman wishes to remain home but cannot for financial reasons, it should be possible for her to receive adequate monetary support, at least until her children reach school age.

● Employers should be encouraged to provide flexible conditions for female workers with children, e.g. facilities for time off during school holidays or if a child is sick. Two women with families holding one job between them has been suggested and can be successful.

## THE EFFECT OF MASS COMMUNICATION MEDIA

Children are exposed to a wide variety of influences through radio, television, films and comics and public concern is often expressed as to the effects of these. Packard (1957) has described how attempts are made to increase sales by advertisements which appeal to children. Violence displayed on television has recently come under fire (*Brit. Med. J.* 1976). Does this produce imitative behaviour and an increase in aggressive behaviour, or does it serve as an escape valve for aggression which cannot be expressed overtly? There is no clear answer, but the lonely, understimulated child is more susceptible than the well adjusted individual.

It seems that different children selectively use whatever is available according to their individual needs. Programme refinement cannot be a substitute for supervision of children's viewing by responsible parents.

## CLINICAL EXAMPLES

*A child's behavioural disturbance reflects her mother's personality disorder*

Jennie was an 8-year-old who showed alimentary rebellion to her mother's coercive management. She vomited when forced to eat and soiled her pants at school. Although the latter probably had as its basis a maturational lag, the smother love to which she was subjected played a major role in perpetuating the disturbance. Jennie weighed 6 stone, mother's 18 stone related in every sense to an overload of conflicts dating back to her childhood. She had been involved in an incessant power struggle with her own mother and found solace in eating. Even at 40 she still resorted to food as a means of 'calming her nerves'. Mother's immature adjustment made it hard for her to give Jennie affection and she assuaged her guilt in relation to this, by equating love and food and feeding her constantly. Since Jennie's appetite was small, there were constant battles at meal times. Jennie stoutly resisted all her mother's attempts to make her conform to being a miniature replica of herself, as a basis for working out her own childhood feelings. Although mother and daughter regularly appeared in identical dress, she did all in her power to alter things. Her encopresis started in the first year of school. Mother was furious. She felt she was losing control of the child, let alone her bowels, and devised various methods of punishment, such as asking the teacher to place erring children next to the smelly Jennie in class. Jennie's fury equalled her mother's. She refused to 'go' at home with a questioning mother standing outside the toilet and the battle of the bowel continued unabated.

### A child's 'symptoms' relate to his mother's depression

Mrs. T. was unable to conceive and had 2 adopted sons. She visited agency after agency complaining that the eldest, Richard, aged 7 years, suffered from bedwetting, and made each visit an opportunity to hint at her husband's liking for female companions and her own symptoms, among which heartburn figured prominently, and in one sense not inappropriately.

She moved Richard from a school near a creek because she felt it was inadequately fenced. She rushed him to hospital saying he had swallowed some bleach. In fact, it seemed highly unlikely he had done so, although he had played with the bottle. Next she complained of his 'stealing', taking lollies from the kitchen. Reassurance produced little effect and there followed a series of visits to hospital because of physical complaints (coughs, colds, diarrhoea and stomach ache), when examination always showed a healthy child.

When Richard's file was three quarters of an inch thick, she reached the end of her tether and Psychiatric Outpatients. She was given an opportunity to talk. She expressed her misery about her inability to have children of her own, and worries lest she was 'not a good enough mother' for Richard. She felt she had lost her husband's affection and would soon lose that of her boys. Questioning revealed the typical symptomatology of depression, with sleep disturbance, loss of weight, anergia and ruminations about the possibility of harm coming to her sons. She was helped by referral for marriage guidance, antidepressants, and supportive care by her family doctor.

## Sociocultural deprivation

Ronald was $9\frac{1}{2}$ when he was referred by his teacher as 'a disruptive influence'. He was considered 'very dull indeed'. He came to the clinic with his grandmother, an old age pensioner who was deaf and vague, nevertheless he appeared very fond of her and repeated the doctor's questions to her, shouting loudly as he did so. His father had been injured at work, was for some reason ineligible for a pension and took light work whenever he could find it. He was away from home for long periods. Mother, a barmaid, was the main wage earner.

His household comprised mother, father, five siblings, two illegitimate children of an older sister, the maternal grandmother and grandfather, and a couple whose identities were dubious and who were called 'uncle' and 'aunt' by Ronald.

After the social worker's first visit to the home she reported: 'The family live in a dilapidated, untidy, wooden house which is not weatherproof. There are 3 bedrooms and 4 beds which older members of the household appear to occupy in turn. The children are relegated to 'divans' on the verandah. Mother, father and 3 older siblings were at home away from work, 'recovering' from a wedding party'.

Her second visit gave cause for much thought. She met a policeman on the doorstep who was making enquiries about goods missing from a nearby warehouse. After he had left she was offered as a gift, an expensive bottle of perfume. On the third visit, during school hours, the 3 younger children were home alone, with Ronald in charge. The house was dirty and very cold. The children said that grandmother was ill and mother had been off work. There seemed to be little food about and the children explained a man had come and taken away their television set.

Ronald's teacher was young and keen, but had little appreciation of the difficulties under which many of the families in the neighbourhood laboured. Ronald's attendance record was erratic. When in class, he spent much time teasing other children and acting the clown. He was often poorly and unsuitably clad and known to steal from his classmates' lunch boxes. In the playground he was fiercely protective of his sister's two children. The staff noted his grandmother's propensity to wait at the school gates on the days when her pension was paid and 'treat' the children, Ronald especially, on their way home. Although psychological assessment showed that Ronald was only slightly below average intelligence, his reading age was 3 years behind his chronological age and he had mastered only a few basic skills in mathematics.

## A child's reaction to parental psychosis

Montgomery was 11 and referred by his school with complaints relating to his effeminate appearance, poor school work, and stealing from female teachers. He put flowers on his desk and in his buttonhole and lipsticks had been found in his pockets. School work had become increasingly poor over the past 2 years. Unless closely supervised he would spend his time in class drawing, painting and writing simple little poems.

His mother came from an 'artistic and spiritualistic' family and reported that Montgomery was the son of her 'spiritual guide', a man killed in World War II with whom she communicated regularly and who directed her actions. When she was aged 30 he suggested to her that she should have a child. She went abroad, met a man whom she said she knew for a couple of weeks and who left her pregnant with Montgomery. Montgomery, named after this 'spiritual' father, had been reared in the belief that he was his son. His babyhood was disturbed by mother spending periods in a psychiatric hospital. On her return home she married a man much older than herself who drank heavily and was at times violently abusive toward Montgomery and herself. Montgomery slept in his mother's bed, the step-father was relegated to an outhouse known euphemistically as the studio.

On examination Montgomery was ethereal and effeminate. He was terrified of his step-father and spoke of the harsh treatment he had received. When questioned about his natural father, he said, "Oh, he was killed in France in the war", then corrected himself with embarrassment, 'I mean in a car accident'. He appeared to have partly accepted his mother's delusional ideas relating to his birth, but had a sufficient grasp of reality to question them (he was seen in 1975). When asked about his mother's statement that he conversed with spirits and they helped him with homework (apparently unsuccessfully) he became defensive and silent. Psychological assessment showed a boy of normal intelligence whose verbal ability was somewhat advanced for his age. Projective testing showed no strong male identification and he gave his favourite occupations as painting, growing flowers and knitting.

Obviously this boy was in precarious balance, both as regards reality testing and sexual identification. In view of the extremely threatening figure presented by his step-father, it is not surprising he retreated into a feminine role.

Montgomery's mother was persuaded to visit a psychiatric clinic again, and he was for a time admitted to a residential school, where he began to adopt more masculine behaviour. However, after some months his mother took him to another part of the country and contact was lost.

### A child's reaction to his parent's drug addiction

Peter was the 9-year-old illegitimate son of a woman with a history of several admissions to psychiatric hospitals for drug abuse and alcoholism. During his mother's absences he had been cared for in a State institution but had been discharged in his mother's care several months previously, with the proviso that she took him regularly to a children's clinic. These attendances lapsed and a reminder was sent. He arrived at the clinic with his mother, who was obviously under the influence of drugs. Peter pushed her up the steps, found a chair for her and extinguished her cigarette when she fell asleep, her hand drooped, and her coat started to burn.

He answered questions cheerfully, realistically and in a surprisingly mature fashion. He collected the pension, did the shopping, cleaned, washed and ironed after school, and locked up at night to protect her from the unwelcome advances of the man next door.

When it was suggested to him that he might be more happily occupied in playing with his friends, he disagreed. He knew it was important to keep himself and the home looking tidy. He was afraid 'the Welfare would get him', if this was not done.

### Child abuse

A 9 months-old-girl was admitted to hospital having been thrown across a room by her mother. She was covered with bruises and X-ray revealed a greenstick fracture of her left humcrus. The brother, the only other child in the family had been in the same hospital 3 months before having ingested several tablets of aspirin, and with an infected rat bite on his back.

The mother said she had never felt secure or wanted. Her own parents had separated during her infancy and she was reared in an orphanage. At the age of 12 she went to a foster home, then because of disciplinary problems, to a remand home. In adolescence she had several admissions to a psychiatric unit associated with suicidal behaviour which appeared to be motivated toward drawing attention to herself. She functioned in the borderline range of intelligence and had a very poor school record. At 17 she was 'forced into marriage' with a man 12 years older. He showed little interest in his home or children and spent a large proportion of his earnings on gambling and drank heavily. The family were badly in debt.

This is how the mother described her attack on the child:

'We were living in this terrible place; when it rained, water came right up the steps and I couldn't let the children out. Both kids had colds and were crying a lot. Jack (her husband) was worried about work, because some of his mates had been put off. He came in one night and couldn't stand the racket so he went back to the pub and came home "full". He wanted to have sex with me but I wouldn't, I was tired and I made so much noise fighting him it woke Debbie and I was up most of the night settling her. Next day I felt terrible. Gary (the brother) ran out twice and some people brought him back and said I shouldn't let him wander near the road like that. Then Debbie started crying. I gave her a bottle but she wouldn't suck. I couldn't stand it any longer. I just threw her across the room. She lay very still and I said "My God, I've killed her". Then Gary came in and I pushed him out with a brush. Debbie started to cry again so I knew I must get her to hospital but I thought I'd get sent to gaol for what I'd done. When I got there I told the doctor Gary had done it with a brush but he said "come on you must tell me the truth", so I told him what happened.'

This mother agreed to her children being placed in a children's home while arrangements were made to improve the conditions under which she was living. She visited the children daily and formed a very good relationship with the hospital social worker. Help with debts and housing, contraceptive advice, and finding the father more stable employment did much for this couple and after 6 months the children were returned to them. The social worker maintained close contact with the family for the following year. During this time it was noted that both parents, especially the mother, matured considerably. It was the mother's suggestion that this case be made available for others to read. She hoped parents in a similar situation would learn that help was available.

# BIBLIOGRAPHY

## ADOPTION

### References

BRIT. MED J. (1977) Editorial. *Adoption of Deprived Children.* **2**, 280–81.
SEGLOW J., KELLMER-PRINGLE M. & WEDGE P. (1972). *Growing up Adopted.* London, National Foundation for Education Research in England and Wales.
WOLFF S. (1973). Illegitimacy and family disruption. In *Children Under Stress.* Ringwood, Victoria. Penguin Books Australia Ltd. p. 129.

### General reading

KORNITZER M. (1959). *Adoption.* London, Putnam. (A book addressed to English parents).
MED. J. AUST. (1972). *Editorial.* Adoption, **2**, 1098–1099.
MCWHINNIE A.M. (1967). *Adopted Children, How They Grow Up.* London, Routledge Kegan Paul.

## BEREAVEMENT IN CHILDHOOD

### References

BROWN F. (1961). Depression and childhood bereavement. *J. Mental Sc.*, **107, 754.**
GREER S. (1964). The relationship between parental loss and attempted suicide. *Brit. J. Psychiat.* **110**, 698–705.
RUTTER M. (1966). *Children of Sick Parents.* Maudsley Monograph No. 16. London, Oxford University Press.

### General reading

ANTHONY S. (1973). *The Discovery of Death in Childhood and After.* Ringwood Victoria, Penguin Books Australia Ltd.
BROWN F. (1968). Bereavement and lack of a parent in childhood. In *Foundations of Child Psychiatry.* E. Miller (ed.). London & New York, Pergamon Press.

### Books which may be used to introduce children to the concept of death

BROWN M. (1965). *The Dead Bird.* Addison-Wesley, Young Scott Books.
SHECTER B. (1973). *Across the Meadow.* Garden City, New York, Doubleday.
SONNEBORN R. (1971). *I Love Gran.* New York, Viking Press.
FASSLER J. (1971). *My Grandpa Died Today.* New York, Behavioural Publications.
CAINES J. (1973). *Abby.* New York, Harper & Row.

# ILLEGITIMACY

*Reference*

LANCET. (1972). Editorial. *Born illegitimate.* **1**, 362.

# PARENTAL DIVORCE

*References*

BRIT. MED. J. (1972). Editorial. *The plight of one parent families,* **2**, 667–668.
BROWN F. (1968). *Prevention of Damaging Stress in Children.* London. Churchill.
GOLDSTEIN J., FREUD A. SOLNIT J. (1973). *Beyond the Best Interests of the Child.*
    New York, Free Press.
McDERMOTT J.F. (1970). Divorce and its psychiatric sequelae in children. *Arch.
    Gen. Psychiat.* **23**, 421.

*General reading*

BRIT. MED. J. (1971). Editorial. *Children of divorce,* **1**, 302.
SCHLESINGER B. (1976). Divorce & Children, a review of the literature. *Reports of
    Family Law* **24**, 203–216.

# PSYCHIATRIC DISTURBANCE IN PARENTS

*References*

ANTHONY E.J. (1969). Clinical evaluation of children with psychotic parents
    *Amer. J. Psychiat.* **126**, 2, 177–184. (*Annual Progress* Vol **3**, 1970).
RUTTER M. (1966). *Children of Sick Parents.* Maudsley Monograph No. **16**.
    London, Oxford University Press.
WOLF S. (1973). Chapter **7**, The neurotic family. in *Children Under Stress.*
    Ringwood, Victoria, Penguin Books Australia Ltd.
WATTS C.A.H. (1966). *Depressive Disorders in the Community.* Bristol, John
    Wright & Sons Ltd.

# SOCIAL FACTORS

*References*

BRIT. MED. J. (1976). Editorial. *Children who die through social disadvantage,* **2**,
    962–3.

BRIT. MED. J. (1976). Editorial. *Violence and television.* **1,** 856.
WALLSTON B. (1973). The effects of maternal employment on children. *J. Child Psychiat. and Psychol.* **14,** 81–95. (*Annual Progress* Vol **6,** 1974).
PACKARD V. (1957). *The Hidden Persuaders.* Ringwood, Victoria, Penguin Books Australia Ltd.

## General reading

HELLMUTH J. (1968). *The Disadvantaged Child.* New York, Brunner Mazel.
ROWLEY C.D. (1972). *The Remote Aborigines.* Ringwood, Victoria, Penguin Books Australia Ltd.

## VIOLENCE TO CHILDREN

### References

BIRRELL R.G. & BIRRELL J.H.W. (1968). The maltreatment syndrome in children, a hospital survey. *Med. J. Aust.* **2,** 1023–1029.
BRANT R.S.T. & TISZA V.B. (1977). The sexually misused child. *Am. J. Orthopsychiat.* **47,** 1, 80–90.
BRIT. MED. J. (1972). Editorial. *Incest and family disorder.* **2,** 364–365.
DALTON K. (1975). Paramenstrual baby battering. Letters to the Editor, *Brit. Med. J.* **2,** 279.
KEMPE C.H., SILVERMAN F.N., STEELE B.F. (1962). The battered child syndrome. *J. Am. Med. Assn.* **181,** 17–24.
KEMPE C.H. (1973). Practical Applications. The abused child & rehabilitation of abusing parents. *Paediatrics.* **51,** 804–812.
LUKIANOWICZ N. (1972). Incest. I. Paternal incest., II. Other types of incest. *Brit. J. Psychiat.* **120,** 301–313.
LYNCH M.A., ROBERTS J. & GORDON M. (1976). Child abuse early-warning in the maternity hospital. *Dev. Med. Child Neurol.* **18,** 759–766.
OLIVER J.E. & TAYLOR A. (1971). Five generations of illtreated children in one family pedigree. *Brit. J. Psychiat.* **119,** 473–80.
RENVOIZE J. (1975). *Children in Danger.* The Causes and Prevention of Baby Battering. Ringwood, Australia, Penguin Books Ltd.
RESNICK P.J. (1969). Child murder by parents. *Amer. J. Psychiat.* **126,** 325.
ROGERS D., TRIPP J., BENTOVIM A., ROBINSON A., BERRY D. & GOULDING R. (1976). Non accidental poisoning: an extended syndrome of child abuse. *Brit. Med. J.* **1,** 793–796.
SCHMITT B.D., KEMPE C.H. (1975). The paediatricians role in child abuse and neglect. *Current Problems in Paediatrics.* L. Gluck, Ed-in-Chief. Chicago Ill. *Year Book Medical Publications* **5,** 5, 3–47.
SCOTT P.D. (1977). Non-accidental injury to children. *Brit. J. Psychiat.* **131,** 366–800.
SMITH S.M., HONIGSBERGER L. & SMITH C.A. (1973). E.E.G. and personality factors in baby batterers. *Brit. Med. J.* **2,** 20–22.

*See Appendix B.

General reading

BESWICK K., LYNCH M., ROBERTS J. (1976). Child abuse and general practice. *Brit. Med. J.* **2**, 800–802.
HELFER R.E. & KEMPE C.H. (1968). *The Battered Child.* Chicago, University of Chicago Press. (This contains a chapter describing a psychiatric study of parents who abuse their children).
KEMPE C.H., HELFER R.E. (1972). *Helping the Battered Child and His Family.* Philadelphia, J.B. Lippincott Co.
MED. J. AUST. (1974). *Editorial.* The battered baby syndrome: some practical aspects. **2**, 231–232.
MED. J. AUST. (1977). *Editorial.* Child Abuse **2**, 619–620.

*See Appendix ii.

# Chapter 7
# How Children React to Stress

'I'm very brave generally', he went on in a low voice,
'Only today I happen to have a headache'. (Tweedledum)

Lewis Carroll (Charles Lutwidge Dodgson).
1832–1898.

We have looked at situations which are stressful for children; how children react to these will be considered next. A child s response to adverse circumstances will be determined by his innate constitution, his previous life experiences and the example set by significant figures in his environment. If the child is handicapped in any way, for example if C.N.S. function is impaired, then he is likely to show increased vulnerability to stress, so will the individual who has been encouraged to remain excessively dependent upon his parents. Thus on one hand there is the robust personality who can take most life events in his stride, on the other, one who reacts to even minimal stress with emotional disturbance. Such disturbance may be expressed through physiological malfunction and situations where this occurs will be examined in Chapter 8. Here we will look at the child's psychological responses to stress.

## TYPES OF RESPONSE – NOMENCLATURE

*Emotional disturbance* is a term which has come into popular use and is generally taken to cover any disturbance not primarily due to organic brain disease. Since emotional disorders in childhood do not fit easily into categories of emotional illness in adults (neurosis) and there is little continuity between emotional disorder in childhood and neurosis in adult life it has been suggested that a category 'disturbance of emotions specific to childhood and adolescence' be included within the general classification of childhood disorders described in Chapter 3 (Rutter *et al.* 1975). This would include:

- states of anxiety
- states of misery
- states characterised by shyness and withdrawal.

States characterised by anger and aggression might be added but it should be realised that the angry child is an anxious child since he fears being overwhelmed by his aggression, as well as retaliation by the object to whom his aggression is directed. However it is still accepted that neurosis can be recognised in childhood: with this in mind we will look at the manifestations of anxiety in childhood, transitory responses to stress (adaption reactions) neutotic disorders (which represent a more severe degree of pathology) and finally long-standing problems of personality and the behaviour which goes with them and which may merit the term 'personality disorder' even in childhood.

## THE ANXIOUS CHILD

Anxiety is an appropriate reaction to situations which involve physical danger or psychological stress. Some children, however, are brought for advice because they are in a continuous state of nervous tension. They over-react to situations which peers take in their stride, e.g. school tests or mother leaving home for the day, as well as to those which could normally be counted on to produce anxiety such as a change of school, or going into hospital.

The contribution made by heredity to this clinical picture is unknown but most of these patients come from anxiety-ridden backgrounds and parental example is important.

### *Symptoms*

Direct manifestations:
● The child subjectively experiences anxiety. Since 'anxiety' is not commonly in a child's vernacular, he will say he feels 'awful' or 'scary'.
● Physiological manifestations associated with autonomic over-activity i.e. frequency of micturition (sometimes bedwetting), diarrhoea, nausea, vomiting, and sleep disturbance are all common and may be the reason for bringing the child to attention.
● Appetite is commonly affected, a tense child may eat very little but this is not always the case, and overeating leading to obesity is not uncommon.
Indirect manifestations:
● Behaviour may be clinging, dependent and infantile. Sometimes this is associated with an aggressive element, the child punishing his mother by 'bad' or 'babyish' behaviour as he attempts to gain her attention in order to feel secure.

● School performance is often poor. This may be associated with frequent absences because of somatic complaints or the child may be too involved with his worries to compete with others, or indeed to enjoy life at all. School refusal may develop.

● Irritability is common with inappropriate displays of aggression.

● Attempts to bolster self-confidence may result in antisocial behaviour or acts of bravado, e.g. playing chicken.

## *Management*

Many individuals cope with high levels of anxiety without undue restriction of interests and activities. However, if a child's anxiety is such that it handicaps him in daily life or causes distress to those about him, or both, then it is obvious that something must be done to help him.

Careful assessment of the total situation is necessary. Undue academic pressure, a handicapped sibling or depressive illness in a parent commonly produce anxiety in childhood. It goes without saying that the family doctor is in a strategic position both to assess the child's environment and to offer advice as to how to alleviate the pressures on him. Such advice may be all that is necessary. Sometimes a parent may require help in his own right. An excessively anxious child needs assistance in coming to terms with his difficulties and mastering them. If old enough and verbal enough, this can be done by talking through his problems with an adult. If not, play therapy may be used to allow him to ventilate his anxieties and to demonstrate to him how he can cope with them.

Drugs have a small part to play in management. It is generally better for a child to learn to master his anxiety with the help of a supportive adult than by the use of medication. A tranquilliser such as diazepam may sometimes be necessary on a short-term basis, but should always be regarded as a temporary expedient.

## ADAPTION REACTIONS

Because of the child's sensitivity to environmental events transitory responses to stress are common and adaption reactions are frequently diagnosed in Child Psychiatric practice. They include a wide spectrum of disturbance involving emotions and/or behaviour which would not be expected in a normal child. However, there is no significant distortion of personality development, and the disturbance settles as the stress eases or the child matures sufficiently to be able to cope with it. These reactions are *reversible* and *situation specific*. Before a given stress is blamed for emotional disturbance it must be shown that:

● It was meaningful for the individual.

● There was a time relationship between its occurrence and the onset of disturbed behaviour.

It is all too easy to find possible adverse factors in any environment. The importance lies in determining their effect upon the child.


## NEUROSIS IN CHILDHOOD

Neurotic disorders are characterised by *abnormalities of feeling and behaviour which are not accompanied by the subjective distortions of reality* seen in the psychoses. The neurotic individual is *abnormally sensitive to stress* and he responds to it with an exaggeration of the feelings we all experience at times. Thus there may be anxiety or depression, disproportionate to life events; in addition obsessions, compulsions, phobias and 'hysterical' symptoms may develop as exaggerations (often gross) of behaviour utilized in an effort to control anxiety.

All neurotic children show anxiety at some time, but not all anxious children are sufficiently disturbed to be labelled neurotic. A child should only be diagnosed as neurotic if:

● he becomes morbidly anxious in response to stress, which is often minimal or inapparent to the observer;

● his anxiety is persistent, long standing, and handicaps him in day to day living;

● he shows types of behaviour utilized by neurotic adults in attempting to control anxiety.

Thus, he will show symptoms of anxiety described above plus behaviour indicative of the use of psychological manœuvres (defence mechanisms), in an attempt to cope with anxiety. These defence mechanisms will be considered briefly before describing the symptomatology of the neurotic child.


### Defence mechanisms

Faced with conflicts and the anxiety which accompanies them, the personality looks for ways of defending itself, and a series of mental mechanisms are described which serve this purpose. These are not selected consciously; they become habitual because they have proved effective in the past. It is quite normal to use such defences but neurotic disturbances are characterised by an excessive use of them; the predominant ones selected determine the clinical picture. Common defence mechanisms are: *Repression*, in which anxiety-arousing ideas or wishes are pushed into the unconscious, i.e. selectively 'forgotten'. Although the individual cannot recall the repressed material, this does not mean its influence is absent from the personality. A child may 'forget' a frightening experience but none the less remains timid and fearful.

*Regression* is very common in childhood. The individual reverts to an earlier developmental stage in order to conserve mental energy, e.g. the child who responds to a sibling's birth with infantile behaviour.

*Denial*, in which experience is falsified in order to allay anxiety, is also common in childhood, e.g. quarrelling parents may be represented to the doctor as getting on well.

*Displacement*. Here feelings directed toward a person or object are shifted to another who is less likely to retaliate, and less threatening, e.g. a child who cannot express hostility he feels for his father, becomes aggressive toward his brother.

*Projection*, in which one's own unacceptable feelings are attributed to another, e.g. a child who is afraid to admit his hatred for a teacher reports, when he gets home, that teacher hates him.

*Reaction formation*. The individual assumes attitudes which are diametrically opposed to unacceptable wishes and fantasies, e.g. the child who shows excessive concern and solicitude for a demanding and difficult grandparent.

*Ritualistic behaviour*. Attempts are made to control impulses which generate conflicts and anxiety by stereotyped patterns of behaviour, e.g. a child whose sexual curiosity has been aroused by the behaviour of an adult, adopts repetitive patterns of behaviour such as continually counting objects in order to keep thoughts which he has been taught are 'dirty' out of his mind.

*Rationalisation*. The individual attempts to justify unacceptable thoughts by employing pseudologic, e.g. the child who explains his failure to give a disliked younger sibling a present on the grounds that it might 'spoil' him.

Repression and regression are much in evidence in most neurotic illness. Depending upon other mechanisms utilized, so the symptomatology will vary. Thus:

● If reaction formation and ritualistic behaviour are used, then obsessive/compulsive behaviour will be evident.

● If displacement and projection are used, phobic symptoms (illogical fears) will predominate.

● Conversion reactions, where psychological conflicts are converted into somatic symptoms, involve the mechanisms of denial and displacement. In the evolving personality of the child, these mechanisms are still developing and therefore less effective and the utilization of one after the other (as if trying them out to see which is most effective), results in *symptom shift*. Thus, the clinical picture is generally one of mixed neurosis, with phobic, obsessional, conversion and depressive symptoms intermingled, or first one type of symptom may be in evidence, then another.

### *Acute anxiety attacks*

Upon a background of continuous anxiety some event may precipitate an acute reaction when defences prove inadequate and the child becomes panic stricken. Common precipitating factors are hospitalization, or the sudden death of a relative. Anxiety attacks may be misdiagnosd because attention is paid to physiological aspects only, e.g. the rapid pulse rate or hyperventilation and the problem escalates as the child responds to adult anxiety about his physical condition.

### *Obsessive/compulsive behaviour*

Obsessions are thoughts which keep obtruding into consciousness against the individual's will and may be accompanied by compulsions to perform certain acts such as repeated hand-washing. Children go through a phase of obsessional type behaviour in the early school years. Most of us will recall our habit of touching every third railing or walking in the middle of the pavement squares, as did Christopher Robin. This behaviour is usually outgrown, but should it continue and the child persistently use it as a defence against anxiety, the rudiments of an obsessional disturbance may be laid down. An obsessional child usually comes from a compulsive, perfectionistic family. Obsessional neurosis not uncommonly starts in early adolescence; Pollitt's (1957) study of individuals suffering from obsessional illness showed that 68% suffered their first attack before 25, and some individuals began as early as 6-years-old. Occasionally a schizophrenic illness in adolescence in preceded by obsessional symptoms.

### Phobic reactions

A phobia is an irrational fear of an object or situation, recognised as unwarranted by the individual, who is nonetheless helpless to overcome it. It represents the displacement of anxiety on to a specific object or situation. Thus, if the phobic object is avoided, so is the anxiety. 'Phobias' are described as part of the developmental progress of young children, and may be quite common between the ages of 3 to 6 years, when fear of animals or of the dark is not unusual. Normally such fears are outgrown by the middle school years. It is sometimes hard to determine to what extent a fear is pathological, however, an example will illustrate the difference.

● A school age child who dislike dogs, and is uneasy if one is around, could be considered normal; but if he becomes preoccupied with meeting one and is in a constant state of anticipatory anxiety, then he could justifiably be regarded as phobic.

School phobia will be discussed later in this chapter (see p. 110).

### Depression

Many unhappy children referred for help, show a disturbance which could reasonably be expected in their particular situation. Depression is only diagnosed when the disturbance is *out of proportion* to the precipitating factors and parents describe a *persistent and pervasive change in mood.* The occurrence of depressive illness in childhood has only recently been recognised, because somatic or behavioural symptoms are often so prominent that the underlying affective disturbance is missed.

Infants separated from parent figures fail to thrive and show delayed psychological development in spite of adequate physical care. Psychoanalytic writers have equated this condition with depressive states of later life and labelled it 'anaclitic' depression (anaclisis = dependence on another for emotional support). While it is quite probable that breaking the child-parent bond may sensitise the individual to loss and predispose him to over-react to real or perceived loss in later life, depressive symptoms as such are not commonly described until middle childhood. By this age they are recognised in three areas:

● *Psychological manifestation.* The child is moody and irritable, and sometimes described as suffering a change in personality. He is anergic, weeps easily, school performance falls off, he loses interest in hobbies and withdraws from the company of friends. Morbid interests, or worries about the safety of others, may develop. A poor self concept is expressed, e.g. 'I'm the dumbest in the class', or 'the ugliest'.

● *Somatic symptoms.* Headache and abdominal pain are common complaints. Sleep disturbance may occur; generally the child is unable to settle at night, is restless and has frightening dreams. Appetite may be reduced, but sometimes the child overeats in an effort to compensate for his unhappiness.

● *Aggressive behaviour.* Some children express the misery they feel through antisocial acitivity. Stealing is particularly common. Senseless acts of vandalism, especially fire setting, may occur.

Depressive illness usually appears as part of a neurotic disturbance in childhood, however it may follow a viral illness even in a previously well adjusted child (see p. 138). It is doubtful whether depression in childhood ever reaches psychotic proportions.

The effects of bereavement are described in Chapter 6. Depression and suicidal behaviour in adolescence in Chapter 12.

## Conversion and dissociative reactions

The term 'hysteria' is loosely used, often in a derogatory way and has been replaced by two categories of psychological disturbance.

● *Conversion reactions* where neurotic anxiety is expressed through physical symptoms which are generally in the somato-sensory system i.e. voluntary musculature and sensory system.

● *Dissociative reactions* in which anxiety-loaded thoughts are cut off from the mainstream of mental functioning and pushed out of awareness. Sometimes a sudden and massive loss of memory may occur, and the individual is found wandering in a trance-like state, or fugue. These states are not common in childhood, but become more frequent as adolescence approaches.

Typically when conversion symptoms develop there is a reduction in anxiety (primary gain) and the patient may show an attitude of unconcern – la belle indifférence – however in childhood anxiety often remains prominent. Conversion reactions may be quite transient in childhood and commonly involve limb paralyses or visual disturbances. One 8-year-old progressed from diplopia to seeing six objects when one was held in front of her, during a series of examinations. However, a wide variety of somatic disturbances may occur and sometimes be suggested by illness in a member of the child's family. Functional prolongation of symptoms following physical illness can be very puzzling to the doctor and are not uncommon if the child is rewarded for being an invalid (secondary gain) or the anxious physician chases too actively after the rare and the obscure ordering a plethora of laboratory investigations on a suggestible child (the thick file syndrome). Conversion symptoms are recognised by their non-anatomical distribution and their relationship with emotionally disturbing events.

## *Treatment*

The management of *anxiety* in childhood has already been discussed. Careful appraisal of the child and his family is essential. Since neurosis often relates to family disturbance, it may be necessary to treat a parent concurrently or the family as a unit (family therapy). Overall, treatment involves environmental manipulation and placing the child in a psychotherapeutic setting (group or individual) which allows him to ventilate his feelings and work through his difficulties. Drugs are occasionally needed to reduce anxiety while other measures take effect, e.g. the child who presents on the eve of an examination when there is no time for psychotherapeutic measures to be instituted. It should never be suggested that drugs offer a solution to emotional problems. The child should be told that he is being given medication to make the situation more tolerable while he faces up to his difficulties. *Obsessive/compulsive symptoms* should be accepted without comment. Parental criticism and perfectionistic standards must be eased. Hobbies and interests involving physical activity and sport should be encouraged especially if this involves the child getting away from a home where obsessive standards pertain. *The phobic child* needs an opportunity to talk about his fears. Behaviour therapy which involves the principles of relaxation and deconditioning may be used. *Conversion symptoms* can usually be removed by suggestion, demonstrating to the child that he can use the affected part normally. Placebos, 'magic', ridicule and criticism have no part to play, but a careful explanation of how emotional difficulties can affect function, has. Restoring normal function is only half the management. Investigation of underlying difficulties which are often associated with family attitudes is essential. *Depression* generally responds to modification of the environment, supportive help, and an opportunity for the child to express his misery and the aggression which is closely associated with it. Any suggestion of self-destructive behaviour should be taken seriously, and admission to hospital may be warranted. If the condition seems persistent and long-standing, the tricyclic antidepressants may be necessary (see Appendix A).

## SUMMARY

It is reasonable to postulate a continuum involving the disorders described above. At one end is the *normal child* whose response to adverse environmental happenings is appropriate and proportionate to their magnitude. Next come children who show a degree of disturbance outside the limits of normal but this is transitory and settles quickly when the stress is removed (*adaption reactions*). At the other end is the child who is unduly vulnerable and shows *neurotic disturbance* even when stress is minimal.

## THE CHILD WHO IS FREQUENTLY ABSENT FROM SCHOOL

This is a major problem with education authorities and one in which the doctor is commonly involved since he must decide when a child should return to school after illness and may be consulted about emotional disturbance reactive to school difficulties.

The reasons for repeated absences or a long period away from school are:

### *Chronic physical illness*

Naturally this accounts for many absences. However, if the child or his mother are averse to regular school attendance it is surprising how often symptoms become accentuated or prolonged after the physical basis for them has resolved.

### *School and family problems – reality factors*

Migrant children with social difficulties, and children with learning problems, may well find excuses for not going. So may parents who need the child at home, to mind a shop or young siblings. These reasons for non-attendance are understandable, and can be dealt with on their merits.

## Truancy

These children, generally older boys, 'disappear' on the way to school, or immediately following roll call, and roam the streets all day, often in the company of others and return to tell their parents they have been at school. They are poorly motivated toward school work, as are their families and often show antisocial behaviour generally. Medical treatment has little to offer. They are better dealt with by education authorities, social agencies or sometimes the police.

## School refusal

In this group the reasons for non-attendance are harder to understand. Typically a good student, although dull children are not immune, the child says he will go to school, but as the time approaches he becomes anxious and unable to leave home, or if he reaches school, unable to go in. Sometimes he appears panic-stricken, and neither threats, bribes nor punishment have any effect upon him. He returns home and does not leave during school hours. If he gets into school he may settle for the day, but the panic recurs the next morning. Anti social behaviour is remarkable for its absence, and teachers cannot understand why a quiet and conscientious child should fail to attend. Because the child's fear of school seems irrational, 'school phobia' is often used to describe the condition, but in fact the problem stems from anxiety on separating from mother and home, separation anxiety, and the child projects his fears on to the school.

The pattern is one of increasing reluctance to go to school, which gradually progresses to total refusal. Sometimes it is precipitated by an absence from school due to physical illness. By the time they reach the doctor, many weeks of schooling may have been lost. Commonly these children are overprotected and overdependent. Many of the mothers have neurotic difficulties, and cling to the child on school mornings quite as hard as the child clings to them. Commonly mother and child interact together in a vicious circle of hostility and dependence. Ostensibly mother pushes the child to school, covertly she pulls him back and then tells him what a bad boy he is. Although good providers, the fathers are ineffectual and unable to exert firmness, especially at school time.

When it presents a clear cut picture as described, there is no difficulty in recognizing school refusal. However, presenting symptoms are often somatic and the family doctor may be the first to be consulted. Nausea, loss of appetite, vomiting, syncope, headache, abdominal pain, diarrhoea, malaise and even limb pains are common complaints. The absence from school may not even be mentioned unless it is asked for. Close questioning reveals that these symptoms occur only on school mornings and holidays are free of them. One boy who lived opposite his school told the writer his stomach-ache came on half-way across the road. If the child returns home symptoms disappear miraculously; if he is persuaded to remain at school they usually pass off by lunch time. These cases can present difficult diagnostic problems, since aside from the somatic symptomatology the child may give a very plausible reason for non-attendance, for example failure in a specific subject, or a difficult teacher and it is only when a removal of these factors produces no improvement that the true nature of the disturbance is recognized.

*School refusal is not uncommon*, referrals of girls outnumber boys in the early grades, but this is reversed later. There are two peaks of frequency, one at the start of school life, between 5 and 7 years, and the other around puberty and the start of high school. In the younger group, separation problems are obvious. In the older group, there may be indications of serious psychopathology, such as neurosis often with symptoms of depression, personality disorder or, rarely, psychosis.

*Treatment* of school refusal is an urgent matter. Medical mismanagement may result in a potentially reversible disorder becoming a chronic and irreversible mental disturbance. The child must be returned to school. If he is away for even a short time he gets behind with his work, he is isolated from the normalizing influence of his peers and is trapped into closer interaction with a sick family. Therefore:

● He must be given a date to return and no redress be allowed. He must go every day.

● He should not be put on a correspondence course.

● He must not be transferred to another school. If he does he will go for a few days then the problem will recur, and he is less likely to receive help in a school in which he is not known.

● When somatic symptoms are present, a careful physical examination is essential. Remembering that both child and mother are keen to find excuses for missing school, both readily fall in with plans for any hospital referrals. If these are merited, they should be arranged promptly and after school hours if at all possible.

● It is better for someone other than the emotionally involved mother to escort the child to school. If working flexible hours the father may help, or a neighbour may take him.

● Discussion with the school staff will allow help to be given to the child when he arrives. A teacher who is prepared to meet the child at the gates and escort him in can be invaluable. It is wise to make school particularly rewarding for a few weeks, for example by giving the child some extra privileges.

● A tranquilliser such as diazepam can be useful on school mornings in the older child if anxiety is severe. Where drugs are used, the child should be told that he is being given tablets for a short period only to make symptoms become more bearable while he gets himself back to school.

● Return to school does not mean the whole problem has resolved. Work with the family is essential. Child and parents need reassurance as to the absence of physical disease and explanation as to the nature of the symptoms. The child's need for independence must be appreciated by his parents.

*School refusal in older children* may be hard to treat. The onset is often insidious with a history of previous episodes of reluctance or refusal to attend school. Although the principles of management are the same as for the younger child, it can be difficult to implement these in the high school child. Sometimes admission to an inpatient adolescent unit may be necessary. About one third of children with school refusal fail to return (Hersov 1972), and most of these are adolescents close to school leaving age. With these, return sometimes is impossible and an early start to vocational training seems the only answer. Strangely enough, they will often leave home daily for this.

*Summary.* School refusal is a family problem, and commonly involves the general practitioner. Its recognition can be difficult, not only because of the predominance of somatic symptoms, but because the child may project his irrational fear of school on to some aspect which could be reality-based. Early intervention is essential to prevent the child's disturbance from becoming chronic and irreversible. Treatment generally involves other family members.

## PERSONALITY DISORDERS

These involve pathological attitudes, and behaviour patterns which become more or less a way of life. In view of the child's potential for growth and change, it is not usual to diagnose these disorders before late childhood or adolescence. Nevertheless, relatively permanent traits may become apparent in childhood and The Group for Advancement of Psychiatry suggests a descriptive approach for 'character types' in childhood as follows:

| Personality Type | Characteristics |
|---|---|
| Anxious | ● Chronic tension and apprehension. Anxiety is long standing but is not so crippling as in a neurotic child. |
| Compulsive | ● Excessive orderliness and tidiness with rigid and inflexible attitudes. Obsessional thoughts or compulsive behaviour may develop. |
| Histrionic | ● Overly dramatic, suggestible, seductive and egocentric. Girls are more commonly affected than boys. |
| Dependent | ● Helplessness and immaturity, inability to take initiative. |
| Oppositional | ● Aggression expressed by negativism, stubbornness and refusal to co-operate. |
| Overly inhibited | ● Shyness, passivity and marked constriction of personality functioning. |
| Overly independent | ● A drive toward independence is very strong and the child has difficulty in accepting limits. |
| Isolated | ● Withdrawal, detachment and inability to form meaningful, warm interpersonal relationships. |
| Mistrustful | ● Suspiciousness and secretiveness. These are not common in childhood, but may become apparent in adolescence. |
| Tension discharge disorder | ● Poor impulse control, with a tendency to act out sexual and aggressive drives in destructive ways. Two groups are recognised (a) Individuals who show little guilt or anxiety, and have defective conscience formation (impulse ridden personalities) (b) Individuals whose behaviour is engendered by neurotic conflicts and tension. There is evidence of conscience development, but sometimes it is harsh and punitive. |
| Dys-social | ● Antisocial behaviour which deviates from the normal standards of society, but is consonant with the environment in which the child has been reared. |
| Sexual deviations | ● Are not recognised in childhood and rarely in adolescence. |

# DELINQUENT BEHAVIOUR

Many children show episodes of antisocial behaviour; i.e. behaviour which is not up to socially acceptable standards for their mental age, but generally this is quickly outgrown. If however, it is of sufficient degree and persistence to cause disturbance to the environment, the term *conduct disorder* is used. *'Juvenile delinquency'* is used for behaviour which brings the individual into contact with the law or makes him liable to police action.

Delinquency represents a serious social and financial problem to society; it involves aggressive behaviour toward others or their property (vandalism, fire-setting), stealing, truancy, sexual promiscuity and misuse of drugs or alcohol. Delinquency rates are higher in males, but there is some evidence that it is increasing in females, particularly as regards acts of violence. It rises with industrialization and urbanization and is higher in low income, culturally deprived families, but may occur in any social setting. Children from middle class homes often receive preferential treatment by the authorities and this can distort statistics. Children showing delinquent behaviour fall into two groups:

*Antisocial type.* These individuals are always in trouble and have little conscience and no loyalty to anyone but themselves.

*Dys-social type.* These come from amoral or immoral families. They have identified strongly with deviant models and remain consistently loyal to them.

## *Aetiological factors*

*Constitutional or organic.* Long-term studies have shown that antisocial behaviour may become apparent early in life and persist (Robins 1966). To what extent hereditary factors operate in this respect is unknown. It has been suggested that individuals with *chromosomal abnormalities* XXY (Klinefelter's syndrome) and XYY are predisposed to sociopathic behaviour (Swanson & Stipes 1969) but when this does occur it may well be compensatory to a disturbed body image rather than due to inherent drives. *Mentally subnormal* individuals are suggestible and slow to learn the mores of society but there is no inherent reason why they should show antisocial behaviour either. *Head injury or encephalitis* may be followed by disinhibited behaviour sometimes antisocial in character. An association between *minimal brain dysfunction* and delinquent behaviour has recently been stressed (see p. 169). It is easy to see how much of this could be compensatory to frustration because of handicap. The M.B.D. child's impulsivity and social ineptitude predispose to his being labelled 'naughty' or a 'bad influence' in the classroom. *Learning (especially reading) problems* are frequent in delinquents. Although it seems likely that social factors such as unstable home backgrounds and poor teaching in overcrowded schools are common to both conditions, the histories of some individuals suggest that delinquency develops as a maladaptive response to educational failure resultant to organic brain dysfunction.

*Family life.* Absence of parents, lack of affection in the family, poor identificatory figures, inconsistent management, or over-indulgence by parents appear very commonly in histories of delinquent children. Sometimes a parent derives vicarious pleasure from the child's antisocial behaviour and covertly encourages it. Children who are bored and restricted to inner city areas, with little opportunity for creative activity or organised sport, take to antisocial behaviour as a means of obtaining 'thrills' and excitement. The effect of violence shown on T.V. and in children's comics is discussed in Chapter 6.

*Psychiatric disorder.* Neurotic symptoms, often engendering guilt and a need to be punished or frustration in response to rejection by others, may play a considerable part in the genesis of antisocial behaviour. Mixed neurotic and conduct disturbances are commonly recognised. When such cases are studied, it is possible to demonstrate that antisocial behaviour develops as an attempt to defend against neurotic anxiety. Rarely psychosis, may present with antisocial behaviour (pseudopsychopathic presentation).

The above factors are of important theoretical interest, but studies of individual cases usually show the *interaction of several factors*, and the delinquent child emerges as a victim of his environment and is by no means an easy patient to manage.

## Management

Since juvenile delinquency emerges as a *bio-psycho-social phenomenon*, it must be studied and treated from all angles and this involves:

● Careful clinical assessment; the opinion of a psychologist as regards intellectual function and educational achievement, and an appraisal of home background by a social worker are generally necessary at the start.

● Treatment must be adapted to the individual. Generally a system of rewards for mature behaviour is effective. The patient must learn to earn his privileges. The aim must be to help the delinquent build up stable and secure interhuman relationships and a feeling of responsibility for himself and toward society.

● Psychiatric treatment may be indicated after the initial assessment.

● Treatment should be on an outpatient basis if at all possible. Sometimes a parole system may be necessary to ensure attendances. Treatment of the delinquent *and his family* is highly desirable.

● Residential treatment should only be recommended after careful review. Placement away from home is often perceived as rejection, and increases anger and aggression. If removal from home is necessary, close contact must be maintained between the institution treating the youngster and his parents, who must be involved in case work. It is useless returning an individual to the difficulties which generated his delinquency.

● It is wise to define a definite time for his stay, an indefinite stay makes him insecure and anxious.

● After care is essential to prevent relapses, as is satisfactory job or educational placement.

## Prevention

Delinquency is a serious problem. Preventive measures which are of importance are:

● Paying attention to the underprivileged child.

● Attempting to keep families intact, and providing mother substitutes if a mother is unable to care for her child; offering support to families if the father is absent.

● Providing special educational help, before maladapative responses to school problems have become established.

● Improving facilities for recreation in inner city areas.

## Juvenile courts

By the nature of his work, the child psychiatrist is often associated with juvenile courts. His role involves:

● *Evaluation* of the offender with a view to giving an opinion as to why the disturbance occurred and detection of likely aetiological factors.

● *Giving recommendations* as to management of the case and suggesting available forms of treatment.

● *Initiating psychiatric treatment* if appropriate or arranging for it.
● Giving those who work in juvenile courts a general *understanding* of psychiatric disorder in childhood.

It is important for the Children's Court to develop confidence in reports given by the psychiatrist. Such report should be clear and concise and contain neither jargon nor theoretical treatises. They should include a *diagnostic evaluation* with probable aetiological factors, advice regarding overall *management of the case*, and specific details as to where *treatment* can be obtained if, appropriate.

## CLINICAL EXAMPLES

### *Adaption reaction in a 14-year-old boy*

Jim was referred because even an experienced headmaster found the notes he passed round his class sufficiently obscene to be labelled 'to be opened by the psychiatrist only'. He had a mass of untidy hair, thick spectacles, was of short stature, suffered from scoliosis and wore a spinal brace. His protruding teeth were also encased in metal. Speech was indistinct and close listeners were sprayed with droplets of saliva. Jim's father had recently been diagnosed as suffering from inoperable bronchial carcinoma. His mother was quite depressed and had recently started work outside the home. He had no siblings. With the onset of puberty he became more aware of his bizarre appearance. He was called 'spider man' by groups of giggling girls; the one with whom he would have liked to establish a relationship said she 'wouldn't be seen dead with him'. At this stage he learned of his father's illness, and because of involvement in their own difficulties, his parents withdrew their support. He had always been quite an artist and he discovered that – depending on the nature of his subject – he could get some compensation for the insults and rebuffs of the playground. A suitable drawing plus a caption would be eagerly handed round and he became known as the boy who could produce 'the best'.

Jim came for weekly psychotherapy with a sympathetic male therapist. Discussion with his dentist and orthopaedic surgeon resulted in the spinal brace being discarded and a less obvious dental appliance. He was encouraged to join in peer activities outside the home and, became popular in a youth club where his artistic abilities were capitalised in a more socially acceptable way. As his father's death approached, Jim was able to offer his mother some support and in time coped with the bereavement quite realistically.

Follow up after 2 years showed a well adjusted youth who had started apprenticeship as a draughtsman. His appearance had improved somewhat and he had learned to capitalise on his hair and spectacles by adopting a 'studious' pose. His prognosis is good.

### *Neurotic disturbance with conversion symptoms*

Veronica was a 10-year-old with a week's history of blindness in her left eye. She attributed this to knocking her head on a cupboard, but investigation revealed that it coincided with the death of a school friend's brother. A year previously she had developed contractures of both small fingers following minor injuries to her hands. These persisted for several weeks.

Veronica had always been regarded as nervous. She had a history of poor sleep, nightmares, and frequent attacks of headache and abdominal pain when she 'groaned in agony'. Mother and child were frequent visitors to 3 local hospitals, where Veronica had been subjected to extensive physical investigations from time to time.

Veronica's father suffered from a peptic ulcer, was irritable and demanding, and manipulated the family with his symptoms. Her mother suffered from a multiplicity of 'physical' complaints. There was one sibling, an intellectually handicapped and epileptic boy whose fits were a focus of family concern.

Veronica was a bright, dramatic child who said with a smile, 'I've always something wrong with me. When my eye and my fingers were bad, my brother wasn't allowed to hit me.' Psychiatric investigation revealed some of the problems confronting this child, her murderous feelings toward her sibling, and the extreme anxiety she suffered when her friend's sibling actually died. Her blindness precluded both 'seeing' her friend and attending the funeral.

Veronica's vision was quickly restored by suggestion, and with the help of a therapist she came to understand the relationship between her symptoms and the difficulties she was encountering. Work with the family proved difficult, but the parents were persuaded to spend more time with Veronica after arrangements were made for the handicapped brother to spend a holiday away from the family every year, and better control of his fits was achieved.

Follow-up after 3 years showed no further conversion symptoms, but she had missed several exams because of a very dubious menorrhagia, and there was evidence that she was still using physical complaints as a means of evading stressful situations.

## Neurotic disturbance with obsessional features

Mary was a very intelligent 11-year-old girl whose mother brought a list of symptoms as she was afraid details might be forgotten in the heat of the moment.

Mary's troubles had started 2 months before after seeing a film which involved the killing of her parents by an adolescent girl. She began to worry lest she might harm her parents; and this progressed to ruminations about actually killing them. She continually worried about minor 'transgressions', for example, taking an apple from a friend's house, looking at another girl's book during a test at achool. She was unable to sleep at night until she had 'confessed' to her mother. Compulsive symptoms then made their appearance. She continually visited the toilet to 'check' lest she had started to menstruate. She had to wash her hands after each visit; mother reported this occurring up to 50 times a day.

Mary presented as a neat, methodical, over-conscientious individual who worried excessively before classes at school in case she would not 'get the answers right'. The family were visited by a social worker who reported 'The house is excessively tidy, even in the garden not a blade of grass is out of place. Mary's father objects to 'untidiness', picks up crumbs from the carpet before he leaves for work, he checks light switches and taps continually. He is an accountant and well known for his ability to balance everything to the last cent.'

Psychotherapeutic sessions with Mary revealed some of the anxiety she felt in relation to early pubertal changes and her guilt about an interest in boys 'dirty parts'. At the time her troubles started she had been on a family holiday and because of sleeping arrangements had observed her father and her uncle naked.

Mary's progress was followed for 6 months, the normality of her increased interest in sex was explained and efforts were made to develop interests outside the home, particularly those involving unstructured activities (painting, clay modelling and bush walking). Although initially she became quite depressed and spent a short period in hospital after she told her mother 'the world would be better without me', her symptoms subsided. Her prognosis remains uncertain.

## Neurotic disturbance with depressive features

Rupert, a 12.10-year-old, was admitted to hospital with the complaint that he had been 'very nervous' for the past 8 weeks. There had been a similar episode a year previously. He had always been regarded as sensitive and shy. His parents reported 'He doesn't like the roughness of sport and spends most of his time reading. He can't face up to things and sees everything in a morbid light. He worries what we are doing while he is at school, and if we come home late he is sure we have had an accident'.

Although he had never had any serious physical illness, he complained frequently of headaches, stomach pains and inability to swallow hard substances because of a lump in his throat. He would pick the currants out of cakes because they were too hard. He was particularly sensitive to noise, and had on occasion walked out of the classroom, complaining that the noise there made his head throb.

During these episodes of nervousness he became 'moody and irritable' and the symptoms described above were exacerbated. He lost confidence in himself, complained he couldn't do anything as well as his brother, sat whimpering at school and wept openly at home. On one occasion he attempted to swallow a handful of pills (a tranquilliser prescribed for him), and had hinted several times that it would be better for everyone if he was in the crematorium. Sleep became disturbed and fitful. He ruminated continually about accidents he or his family might have.

School work had always been difficult for Rupert, and his depressive episodes appear to have been precipitated by stress in that area. On the first occasion he was kept down a grade, and thus brought into closer competition with his brighter, and aggressive, younger brother. On the second, he attempted exams preliminary to high school and failed miserably. Rupert's parents were first cousins. Mother had been nervous as a child, and father suffered from hypertension with a history of anxiety attacks.

At interview, Rupert presented with a serious face and talked in a monotone. His complaints were of school, teachers shouting at him, and the noise in the classroom which made his head 'feel like bursting'. He often felt 'scary' with shivers down his spine and these feelings were brought on if he went into a strange house or if he found himself in a crowd.

During his hospital stay, Rupert showed a good response to a milieu designed to divert him from his morbid thoughts, arouse his interests and help him with remedial school work. He was prescribed tricyclic anti-depressants. At times he would express hostility toward his younger brother. During one play therapy session he punched a bean bag aggressively, saying it looked like his brother; later he remarked, 'He's probably dead now'. This was used by his therapist to help him realise how immature and destructive his attitudes were. Unfortunately his mother proved far more difficult to work with. She interfered continually with his management suggesting that nobody really 'understood' Rupert. She sat at the bedside exhorting him to be brave when he developed 'throbbing headaches' prior to visiting the hospital school and broke contact shortly after his discharge.

## School refusal

Jennine was an 11-year-old whose mother brought her for advice because of difficulties in getting her to school. She had attended spasmodically throughout the past year and missed 6 weeks completely prior to visiting the hospital. Initially the problem was one of nausea and abdominal pain on school mornings. She was pale, 'dry retched', unable to eat breakfast and mother said, 'she couldn't go into school when she looked so sick'. She also complained of headaches and urinary frequency.

Jennine had to be driven by her mother to school, and on arrival would cling to the car and had to be forcibly removed from it. Although her disturbance related primarily to school, she had latterly developed similar symptoms in relation to Sunday school and was beginning to show reluctance about journeys away from home without her parents. Jennine's mother arranged to do 'tuck-shop' duty in the school twice a week in order to 'keep an eye' on Jennine, and in the second term obtained a minor teaching position which enabled her to visit the school for a further 2 sessions.

The teacher's report described a pupil who was achieving well, who was quiet and conforming and who had few friends. When questioned about her aversion for school, Jennine said that it was because her best friend had left, later because the teacher bullied her and finally because the boys 'looked at her queerly'.

Jennine's father was a public servant 'very tied up' with his work. The family were in comfortable circumstances. She had two brothers much older than herself. Her mother and the maternal grandmother had had similar difficulties in attending school. The maternal grandfather had died just prior to Jennine's birth and mother described herself as being 'highly anxious' about the baby being frail because of all her worry. She was in fact a fretful baby who suffered from eczema and absorbed a lot of her mother's time because of her skin treatment and 'special' diet. She had always been tense and visits to doctors and dentists produced fainting spells.

On examination, Jennine was excessively polite and rather shy, well developed for her age and attractive in appearance. She reported as follows:

'When I get there (school), I feel all funny. I feel as if I don't want to go in. When my friends come out, I don't want to go to them. I feel all scary, all shivers. I can't breathe and I get this sick feeling. Sometimes I have to go to the toilet a lot, it goes right through me.'

When questioned she said she would like to go to school but 'these feelings' stopped her. She said that there was nothing particular about school that was worrying her, but she 'tried to find things so she wouldn't have to go.'

This case was managed as described in the text. The parents were very anxious about underlying physical illness and a paediatric consultation was arranged after school hours. One careful physical examination (which disclosed a normal pubertal girl) reassured them that all was well. Jennine responded to explanation, the encouragement of a teacher at the school gates and 5 mg of diazepam at breakfast time. Work with her mother proved more difficult. She insisted that it was necessary to drive her daughter to school and although she did as she was instructed (left Jennine with the teacher and drove away), she only went round the block, then walked back through the shrubbery, hopefully unobserved, to see if she had gone in. Regular attendance was achieved for the rest of the school year but difficulties recurred after the long summer holiday.

### Tension discharge disorder resulting in delinquency

Peter was 14 years old when he was referred by a juvenile court for psychiatric assessment. He had a long history of misdeeds, particularly car thefts and stealing petrol. His school report stated that he had been expelled from two previous schools and his headmaster described his behaviour thus:

'This boy is a thorough nuisance. There is nothing bad he hasn't tried and his academic record is poor. His teachers have repeatedly reported him for theft, spying on the girls in the toilet, and using obscene language. His aggression in the playground is very noticeable. I fear, unless he receives help of some sort, homicide may be committed.'

Peter's home background was very unsatisfactory. Although his parents had separated 'officially' when he was 5 years old, his father returned from time to time, chiefly following heavy drinking bouts when he needed time to recuperate and an opportunity to extract money from

Peter's mother. The mother had a regular job, and as well as the time away from home this required, spent hours 'visiting friends', with the result that both Peter and the home were neglected.

Peter was an only child and because of his loneliness his mother's sister had taken pity on him, and he had spent several months of every year with her family. This aunt was a shrewd, intelligent woman and this was how she described Peter's character:

'When you compare him with his cousins he is so different. Ever since he was a small child there's been no stopping him. If he wants something he's got to have it, and he doesn't care how he gets it. Bribes and punishment have no effect, he can't learn, you can't get through to him. If he wants something like pocket money he'll be nice to you, but once he's out of your sight, he'll slang you behind your back if it suits him. He flies off the handle so easily you're afraid to open your mouth sometimes, and he goes mad with rage. He half-killed our dog once, then said he was sorry, but hurt it again the next day. I know he's had a bad start, but somehow it seems born in him. When he was living with us it seemed to be his nature.'

Peter was declared 'in need of control' by the court and admitted to a boys' home. After two years he is showing a degree of self-control. However, the staff still complain of his sudden anger and failure to establish satisfactory relationships with others. It is considered that it is likely he will have to remain 'in care' for a considerable period.

Peter's birth and early life showed no abnormalities and he has always been physically healthy. There has never been any suggestion of brain, damage resultant to injury or infection. He is of good average intelligence but educationally retarded. Undoubtedly his parents' personality problems have contributed to his disturbance, but whether this accounts totally for it is uncertain. His physical appearance and his behaviour both suggest a lag in maturation.

## BIBLIOGRAPHY

### References

HERSOV L. (1972). School refusal. *Brit. Med. J.* **3**, 102–104.
POLLITT J. (1957). The natural history of obsessional states. *Brit. Med. J.* **1**, 194–198.
ROBINS L.N. (1966). *Deviant Children Grown Up.* Baltimore, Williams and Wilkins.
RUTTER M., SHAFFER D. & SHEPHERD M. (1975). *A Multi-axial Classification of Child Psychiatric Disorders.* Geneva, World Health Organisation, pp. 39, 59.

SWANSON D.W. & STIPES A.H. (1969). Psychiatric aspects of Klinefelter's Syndrome. *Am. J. Psychiat.* **126,** 6, 814–822.

## *General reading*

BERCZ J.M. (1968). Phobias of childhood. *Psychological Bulletin,* **70,** 694–720. (**Annual progress* Vol **2,** 1969).

BOLTON A. (1972). The anxious child. *Brit. Med. J.* **3,** 690–692.

DUBOWITZ V. & HERSOV L. (1976). Management of children with non-organic (hysterical) disorders of motor function. *Dev. Med. Child Neurol.* **18,** 358–368.

FROMMER E. (1968). Depressive illness in childhood in Recent Development in Affective Disorders. Coppen, A. and Walk, A. (eds.). *Brit. J. Psychiat. Special Publication,* **2,** 117–136.

JUDD L.L. (1965). Obsessive compulsive neurosis in childhood. *Arch. Gen. Psychiat.* **12,** 136–43.

KAHN J.H. & NURSTEN J.P. (1968). *Unwillingly to School.* 2nd ed. London, Pergamon Press.

MALMQUIST C.P. (1971). Depressions in childhood and adolescence. *New Eng. J. Med.* **284,** 887–893, 955–961. (**Annual Progress* Vol **5,** 1972).

ROCK N. (1971). Conversion reactions in childhood. *J. Amer. Acad. Child Psychiat.* 10(1), 65–93. (**Annual Progress* Vol **5,** 1972).

SHAW C.R. & LUCAS A.R. (1970). *The Psychiatric Disorders of Childhood.* 2nd. ed. London, Butterworths. (Chapter 7, Psychoneurosis).

*See Appendix B.

# Chapter 8
# Psychophysiological Disorders.
# Psychological Aspects of
# Physical Disease. Terminal Illness

Christopher Robin
Got up in the morning
The sneezles had vanished away
And the look in his eye
Seemed to say to the sky
'Now, how to amuse them today?'

A.A. Milne.
*Now We Are Six.*

## PSYCHOPHYSIOLOGICAL DISORDERS

Whenever a child is ill, psychological factors are involved to some extent. The idea that disease is 'organic', i.e. due to physical causes, or 'functional', i.e. has a psychological basis, has become outmoded, and we now think in terms of how much each component contributes to the final picture. Physical disease may produce psychological sequelae, e.g. behavioural disturbance resultant to head injury, or psychological disturbance somatic symptoms (functional disorder), e.g. chronic, recurrent abdominal pain in childhood, or physical and psychological factors may contribute actively and concurrently to a disease (Pinkerton 1974) (psychosomatic or psychophysiological disorder) e.g. asthma. Other examples of psychophysiological disorders of childhood are obesity, some cases of failure to thrive, infantile eczema, migraine, ulcerative colitis and the periodic syndrome – recurrent episodes of gastrointestinal upset not associated with infection.

*Psychophysiological disorders vs anxiety reactions vs conversion reactions*

*Psychophysiological disorders* involve the direct expression of anxiety manifest through dysfunction of the autonomic nervous system and are associated with chronic emotional stress. Long standing dysfunction may produce structural changes and sometimes even endanger life. *Anxiety reactions* are global reactions to stress (see p. 105) and differ from psychophysiological disorders in that they do not show persistant and predominant involvement of a single organ system nor do structural changes occur. *Conversion reactions* (see p. 107) involve the somatosensory system (voluntary musculature), and are associated with underlying emotional difficulties. Only as a long term effect, e.g. through the disuse of muscles do structural changes occur. Thus:

● The child who responds to stress situations with asthma suffers from a psychophysiological disorder.

● The child who responds to a traumatic event with severe anxiety accompanied by several transitory physiological disturbances, e.g. tachycardia, vomiting, hyperventilation, from an acute anxiety reaction.

● The child who responds to punishment by a teacher by developing a paralysed leg which does not allow him to walk to school, is suffering from a conversion reaction.

### Stress as a precipitating factor

What types of stress produce these disorders ? Any life history involves a large number of possibilities. Although relationships with parents are often of paramount importance in children, events have profoundly individual meanings to an individual, and what is significant for one child may not be for another. If an emotional basis for an illness is postulated, it is necessary to demonstrate:

● That the event blamed has specific meaning for the individual.

● A temporal relationship existed between the event and the onset of illness.

### Attention getting value of symptoms

Psychophysiological disorders arise as the direct expression of the child's anxiety in response to stress. They are not a device to gain attention. Once the disease has become established, and if the child derives benefit from it, then symptoms may be perpetuated, but this is secondary to the initial problem.

### Management of psychophysiological disorders

Because of the somatic component, these generally present to the family doctor or paediatrician, and parents may be worried if psychiatric referral is suggested. They feel more comfortable with an 'organic' diagnosis, i.e.

an accredited disease with appropriate treatment, and fear that a psychological aetiology reflects on the quality of their parenting. They need careful explanation of the known facts, and time to reorientate their approach. It is ideal if psychiatrist and paediatrician can discuss the management together with them. Parental anxiety in relation to the child's illness must be accepted but they must be helped to see that overprotection may make matters worse, and should not allow the symptoms to become a focus of family attention.

The child himself may benefit from an opportunity to ventilate his feelings about his illness and should be encouraged to discharge emotion through more appropriate channels.

## BRONCHIAL ASTHMA

This is a common and serious disease of childhood, sometimes it may prove fatal. It can result in psychological crippling through restriction of normal childhood activities. During the attack, the basic disturbance is due to spasm of muscles in the walls of small air passages in the lungs, making it difficult for the individual to exhale air and to cough up and expel liquid secretions. These muscles, like those of blood vessels of heart and abdominal viscera, are supplied by the autonomic nervous system.

Asthmatic attacks appear to be precipitated in 3 ways:

● By contact with some substance (*the allergen*) in the environment not normally harmful, but to which the individual is hypersensitive.
● *Infection* in the respiratory tract.
● *Emotional disturbance.*

Individuals vary as to which factors most often produce attacks, but emotional factors play a role in aetiology at least in 50–60% of asthmatics. Much has been written about the dependency of asthmatic children and the aggression they seem unable to display openly toward their overprotective 'smothering' parents. However, it must be remembered that asthma is very frightening and a threat to life. The extent to which family tensions are involved in asthma can often be demonstrated by removal of the asthmatic child to a residential school or convalescent home (parentectomy); the attacks diminish dramatically and may cease, yet the possibility of contact with allergens remains.

In addition to the medical management of the case (removal of allergens, attention to infections, use of drugs), treatment must be directed to help child and parents deal with emotional stress in a more healthy manner. The aim should be that of the child leading as normal a life as possible in spite of his asthma.

## OBESITY

It is estimated that 10–15% of school age children are overweight. Parents worry lest they are suffering from an endocrine disorder, but this is very seldom the case. They are fat because their calorie intake is in excess of their needs. A child is regarded as 'obese' if his weight is 20% above the average for his age. If very obese before 10 years, the prospects of becoming a slim adult are not good.

In some families there is undue interest in food, most members overeat and are mildly obese but generally well adjusted. However, Bruch (1974) has shown the importance of obesity as a symptom of psychological disturbance. Although several factors may be involved, the most important of these is the *misinterpretation of biological cues*. The child fails to recognise that he has had enough to eat, and when unhappy or anxious finds solace in food. Bruch attributes this to faulty learning in infancy. The mother herself responds inappropriately to her child's signals; she gives food when he cries for attention and comforting, and rewards him for eating when he is not hungry.

This occurs typically in a family setting where the mother is over-dominating and the father passive. Both associate weight gain with good health and children are considered 'good' if they eat voraciously. Such children are often insecure, dependent and sometimes unwanted, and have learned to eat in order to gain parental approval. At school where he is ridiculed, the obese child avoids physical activities because of his poor performance and indulges in solitary pursuits such as reading and watching television, and eating. Thus, a vicious circle is established of obesity→ridicule→unhappiness, anxiety and inertia→excessive food→obesity.

Treatment is difficult since the mother often systematically undoes anything the physician achieves. Dieting by itself produces only temporary results. Attention must be directed towards the parents' emotional difficulties as well as to the child's. Appetite suppressants are not recommended in childhood.

## DWARFISM ASSOCIATED WITH EMOTIONAL DEPRIVATION

Emotional deprivation in early life may be associated with stunted psychological development (see Chapter 3) and failure to thrive physically. Although it has been claimed that inadequate calorie intake is the reason for this, investigation shows that food intake is not always deficient (*Brit. Med. J.* 1974). Some deprived children may eat voraciously, stealing food at times, or develop an appetite for unnatural substances (pica), others drink water compulsively. Removal to a more accepting and stimulating environment may result in amazing weight gain in some instances. For example, a 5-year-old whose mother had strongly negative attitudes towards her (her conception related to the last act of a 'father' before he deserted) and who was referred because of taking scraps from school dustbins, doubled her weight after one year in an affectionate foster home.

## CHRONIC RECURRENT ABDOMINAL PAIN

### Prevalence

This is a common complaint among school age children. In the majority of cases, nearly 9 out of 10 (Apley & MacKeith 1968), no underlying physical disease can be demonstrated despite investigations, 'the diversity and ingenuity of which tend to be in inverse proportion to the experience of the investigator' (Dodge 1976). There is, however, very often a history strongly suggestive of a correlation between the symptoms and emotional disturbance and a family pattern of somatic symptomatology associated with stress.

### The child

Typically of primary school age he will have complained of recurrent attacks of abdominal pain for months, sometimes years. He tends to be tense, timid, fussy, and often does not mix well with peers. Expressions of emotional disturbance may be evident, for example, excessive fears, school difficulties not related to low intelligence, and sleep disorders.

### Diagnosis

This must rest not only on a lack of evidence of organic disease, but on positive evidence of emotional disturbance. Of children with an organic basis for abdominal pain, disease of the urinary tract, often with infection superimposed on a congenital malformation, accounts for about one half.

Traditions die hard but the following deserve mention:
● Threadworms do not cause abdominal pain, they are just as common in children with recurrent abdominal pain as those without it.
● Acute mesenteric adenitis causes abdominal pain, but chronic non-specific mesenteric adenitis is a very doubtful starter and is usually regarded as a diagnosis of the destitute.
● The appendix does not grumble, either it screams or remains silent (Apley 1975).
● The further from the umbilicus the child locates the pain, the less likely is it to be functional.
● If the pain wakens the child at night, it is likely to be associated with physical disease unless anxiety causes disturbed sleep and the pain develops subsequently.
    The family doctor is in the best position to elucidate causative factors. He is likely to know if the family make demands which the child is unable to meet, or if they reinforce the child's complaints with fussy over-solicitude.

## *Management*

This should be along the following lines:
● A full *history* is essential, noting indicators of physical disease (for example, frequency of micturition), and emotional disturbance and whether stressful events correlate with attacks of pain.
● A careful *physical examination* is mandatory. Ancillary investigations should be completed as soon as possible and then finished with once and for all. Laboratory investigations repeated to allay the physician's anxiety because he/she cannot accept a functional basis, raise levels of anxiety in child and parents, to whom a battery of tests suggest sinister diseases. In fact the physician may become a pathogen through suggestion, since anxiety aggravates the symptoms. When ordering ancillary tests, the doctor should ask himself whether he genuinely believes these will confirm pathology (suggested by the history), or whether they are being done 'just to exclude' some remote possibility which could have been excluded within reasonable limits by taking a good history. Hospital visits should be arranged after school hours or during holidays. There is no point in suggesting the advantages of being ill.
● *Urine microscopy* and culture of a midstream specimen of urine is essential.
● *The E.S.R.* is useful if infection is suspected. If abnormal, it points to organic disease, but a normal figure does not exclude this.

● A plain *X-ray film* of the abdomen can also be helpful. It will pick up renal calculi, displaced air shadows which could be associated with an abdominal mass and calcification in a túmour. It may serve as a guide for further investigations such as an intravenous pyelogram in some cases.

● Rarely, *occult blood tests* or a *barium meal* may be done to exclude a peptic ulcer.

● *A tuberculin test* will exclude tuberculosis.

● *The parents must not be told there is nothing wrong with the child.* It is patently obvious there is. Both child and parents need reassurance as to the absence of physical disease, explanation that physical symptoms can be associated with emotional disturbance, that psychogenic pain is real and not something to be ashamed of, and help in resolving their emotional or environmental difficulties.

*Prognosis*

In a follow-up study of 30 untreated patients 8–20 years after an initial examination had shown no organic cause for their abdominal pains, Apley found only one-third to be symptom free. Approximately one-third still had recurrent attacks of abdominal pain and in the remaining third, although the abdominal pains had ceased, other symptoms had developed, commonly recurrent headaches. Nearly one half had 'nervous disorders' of one sort or another. On the other hand from 100 patients with abdominal pains who had been given help with their emotional difficulties (largely in a paediatric setting), 80 showed improvement (Apley & MacKeith 1968).

## CHRONIC RECURRENT HEADACHE

This is also common in childhood and a frequent reason for missing school. Apley & MacKeith (1968) studying 80 consecutive referrals to hospital of children with the complaint of headache, found only 4 with a convincing physical cause, and in three-quarters positive evidence of emotional disturbance. Causes of recurrent headache are –

● *Physical factors* (which are rare), e.g. eyestrain due to astigmatism or infection of nasal sinuses, or systemic disturbance associated with renal disease.

● *Migraine.* Here the attack is acute, often follows stressful events, visual prodomata may occur, the headache maybe unilateral and is followed by vomiting. There is often a history of attacks of vomiting and associated metabolic disturbances earlier in life (cyclical vomiting). A positive family history is common.

● *Emotional disturbance*—complaints of headaches are common in tense, unhappy children. Some may be depressed and hypochondrical. There is commonly a family history of 'nervousness', in fact tension headaches have as strong a family incidence as has migraine. The pain is often described as 'bursting' or throbbing, is central or 'all over', and is generally not associated with abdominal upset.

Because of the sinister overtones of intracranial pathology, many doctors worry lest they have missed an 'organic' cause for the headache. An adequate history will generally give clear pointers as to aetiology. Nevertheless thorough and careful physical examination is essential at the start. The management of functional headache is similar to that for functional recurrent abdominal pain.


ACUTE ILLNESS

This always has psychological overtones, with pain, 'pricks' and restriction of activities on one hand, and increased attention on the other. 'Don't be afraid, doctor won't hurt you', is often repeated by parents but it accentuates rather than repels fear by suggesting to the child a doctor's potential for producing pain.


*The child's response*

Obviously this depends upon age. The young child needs (and demands) his mother's constant attention. He regresses to infantile patterns of behaviour and may become whining and manipulative. The older child may worry about the implications of physical disease and about missing important events. Few are too ill to make some capital out of the situation and may be unwilling to give up privileges allowed during illness, when they are better.


*Parents reactions to a sick child*

Richmond (1958) has described the following stages:
1   Denial and disbelief, 'my child can't become ill'.

2 Fear, frustration and guilt. They blame themselves for allowing the child to fall prey to disease.

3 Intelligent enquiry and planning. They face the situation and attempt to make the best of it.

Supportive care given by professional staff will help toward achieving the latter stage and the parents' trust and confidence in them will be transmitted to, and reassure the child.

Overprotective parents regard illness in their child as a major disaster. The child, reflecting his family's high level of anxiety, generally proves a difficult patient, and may develop an unhealthy interest in body functions and pleasure in playing the role of an invalid. Children of rejecting parents generally prove 'good patients'. Illness represents a relief from punishment and criticism and gains them extra attention. Exaggeration or prolongation of symptoms is not uncommon in these children as well.

### The physician's attitude

The management of acute illness in childhood constitutes a large part of paediatric and general practice. However concern with the child's physical condition often causes psychological concomitants to be over-looked. A doctor's first responsibility is, of course, to diagnose the disease and to start treatment, but if he ignores the implications of illness he is only half treating his patient. *It is essential to treat the child as well as the disease.*

## HOSPITALISATION

A stay in hospital is still a common experience in childhood. For younger children especially, it can be psychologically damaging, and disturbances reactive to it persist for months afterwards. Enlightened attitudes have made hospitals less frightening. Parents visit frequently, ward routines are less strict and a child may bring personal belongings with him, e.g., the battered and questionably clean teddy bear; nevertheless, in the urgency of hospital admission, there is a tendency to forget what the event means to a child. Not only is he separated from his family but he has to adjust to an unfamiliar environment, to strange caretakers (among whom there may be frequent changes) and the effects of the illness itself.

### During the first four years of life

The child suffers chiefly from separation from his background. Three phases are described during the process of 'settling' in (Robertson 1970). *Protest* – when he is grief stricken, throws himself about the cot and pushes away any staff who try to comfort him. He seems to have no idea that mother will return and behaves as if she had gone for good. *Despair* which is characterised by apathy and monotonous sobbing. Because he is quieter, it may be mistakenly believed that he has adjusted. *Denial* when he begins to cut himself off from others. He has been so badly hurt by what he feels as desertion by his mother that he will not risk a repeat of what has happened. He shows more interest in his surroundings and a superficial sociability and will go to anyone in a manner atypical for his age ('promiscuous behaviour'). If mother visits, he is aloof and wary, may cling to the ward sister and refuse to go to her. On discharge, he seems not to trust his mother any more, and may take weeks or months to settle back into normal relationships with his family.

'Hospitalism', is a term often found in the literature. It was first used by Spitz to describe the severe delay in physical and psychological development which results from an infant being permanently separated from his mother and reared in an environment lacking in emotional stimulation.

### In middle childhood

Anxieties relate to anaesthetics, operations and the meaning of illness. Hospitalisation may have been used as a threat and, on admission, the child may be puzzled, wondering what he has done to deserve being put there. Children are well aware of the importance of vital organs such as heart or lungs, and may become very anxious if they suspect these are malfunctioning. Misinterpretations of the actions of staff are common. A hypodermic needle is perceived as a dangerous weapon. It is not only the pricks (often recalled as the worst part of a stay in hospital) that are feared, but what might happen afterwards. Fantasies may develop about the needle breaking, causing the child to bleed or altering feelings and behaviour. Some may feel rejected by parents in favour of brothers and sisters at home. From the age of 8 or 9 years there is a growing awareness of what death really means. The presence of a seriously ill child in the ward may cause far more worry to some patients than staff realise.

## *Puberty*

Sensitivity about body development is common and the youngster may be acutely embarrassed when (as is often the case), he is nursed in a ward in which there is little privacy. As the criterion for admission to a Children's Hospital is generally age, a physically advanced child may find himself out of place. The employment of male nursing staff can reduce the embarrassment of a shy, adolescent boy.

## *Children's behaviour in hospital*

Sympathetic management involves learning to recognise signs of distress in children and why some behave as they do. Students should try to put themselves in the child's place as they study paediatric cases, certainly before they become critical of what they consider 'naughtiness' on the child's part.

● *Anxiety* will make a child restless and sometimes unco-operative or clinging and dependent. Physiological changes associated with anxiety, e.g. an increased heart rate, may cause investigations such as an electrocardiogram to be done and aggravate the situation rather than help it.

● *Regression* to babyish, demanding behaviour is common, and well established behaviour patterns such as good manners or toilet training may break down. Self-stimulation by rocking or excessive thumb sucking denotes not only fear, but boredom.

● *Attention getting behaviour* in an effort to boost confidence is also common. The child manipulates the staff with noisiness or whining and may terrify younger children with stories of what goes on in the operating theatre.

● *Depression* may be associated with the physical effects of the illness or result from psychological stress imposed by it. The child becomes apathetic and withdrawn, and loses interest in books and toys.

● *Prolongation of symptoms* after the physical basis for these has gone is quite common or new symptoms may develop, when a suggestible child is placed among sick children, especially if he lacks interests and activities.

# GUIDELINES FOR THE MANAGEMENT OF THE SICK CHILD AND HIS FAMILY

## Hospital or home?

Obviously, the type of illness, geographical considerations and social conditions will be deciding factors, but the age of the child is most important. No child under four should be admitted without very good reason. If it is imperative, every effort must be made to maintain contact with the parents, especially mother. The latter should either be admitted with the child or encouraged to spend as long in the ward as she can. There is no doubt that she is the best person to nurse her sick child; she doesn't demand time off and is with him continuously. In hospitals where mothers assume routine care, not only does the child benefit, but nursing staff find themselves freed from much time consuming work. 'Care by Parents' units are becoming a feature of modern Children's Hospitals.

## Day care

The admission of children to hospital *by day only* in order to allow surgical procedures or medical investigations and/or treatment to be carried out, has much to commend it as a means of reducing the effects of hospitalisation. Most paediatric hospitals are instituting 'day care units' to cater for this service and it is estimated that within 2–3 years as much as 15%–20% of all elective paediatric surgery may be on these lines (Jones 1976). Points in favour of this arrangement are:

● The child does not spend nights away from home.
● Since the mother remains with her child and acts as 'nurse', he can spend as much time as possible on her knee and not behind cot bars.
● The mother becomes more involved in the child's treatment than would be the case if she only came as a visitor to a ward where he was an in-patient.

## Older children

Children reflect anxiety in their attendants and should be approached with an attitude of quiet confidence. Questions should be answered truthfully, without morbid details, and be at a level which the child can comprehend. Students will only learn what children can understand by talking to them. If treatment is going to hurt, the child should be warned. He should not be expected to be stoic beyond his years, otherwise he will suffer not only the pain but from the feeling he has let his attendant down.

## Attitudes of staff

*Scientific discussion around the bed has no place in paediatric wards.* Children comprehend far more than adults realise and may become very frightened by partly understood statements made by staff. They need someone with whom they can discuss worries, and set great store by having 'my doctor' or 'my nurse', or other member of the staff who shows a personal interest in them. Younger patients can be helped to master their anxieties through play with an experienced therapist.

## Avoidance of boredom

Play leaders and occupational therapists have much to offer a child confined to bed. Schooling should not be neglected for the 'long stay' child. Sometimes hospitals have schools attached or Education Departments can help by sending teachers into the wards to supervise work.

## The parents

Time must be given to them. They often feel useless since hospital staff have usurped their positions as caretakers. Involvement in the child's care will counteract this and help them feel they are contributing toward his recovery. If there is a failure in communication between staff and parents, the latter may become hostile and critical since they feel they are being deprived of information to which they have a right. Explanations in language they can understand and someone available to question (no matter how often) about their child's progress, are essential. Parents should be warned that their child may show regressive behaviour after discharge and that providing this is managed with understanding, it will soon settle.

## PLANNED HOSPITALISATION

When the family knows in advance that a child is to be admitted to hospital, much can be done to reduce anxiety. Simple explanation about the reasons for admission, a preliminary visit to the ward and introduction to staff will help. The child can prepare to go, pack his own case and plan what toys he will take. Books are available from which the child may learn what his visit will entail. (See references at the end of this Chapter.)

## PAEDIATRIC–PSYCHIATRIC LIASON

The appointment of psychiatrists to the staff of children's hospitals has now become general. Areas in which the psychiatrist's training is of particular importance are:

● *Diagnosis*, in cases where both physical and psychological symptoms are evident or where it is suspected that somatic symptoms have a psychological basis.

● *Treatment*, especially of psychophysiological disorders and of psychological disturbance superimposed upon physical conditions.

● *Prevention* of the development of attitudes of invalidism by advising on the management of the sick children.

● *Increasing awareness* of situations where the child's emotional adjustment is at risk, and offering suggestions as to how these can be avoided.

## PSYCHIATRIC SEQUELAE TO PHYSICAL ILLNESS

An acute febrile illness may leave a child apathetic and easily fatigued. Viral infections are often to blame, e.g. infectious mononucleosis. Occasionally quite marked depressive symptoms occur (see p. 107). When this happens, it is often hard to know to what extent physical and psychological factors operate. Over-protective parents may encourage 'symptoms' by allowing extra privileges long after these are necessary. Anxious parents sometimes seek one expert opinion after another, without a definite conclusion being reached and may be given conflicting advice. Understandably this raises their level of anxiety further and this is reflected in the child. Thus, imperceptibly, symptoms due to physical illness are replaced by those with a psychological basis. Careful physical assessment is, of course, essential, but after infections have settled the child must be encouraged to resume his former interests and activities and return to school promptly (see p. 110).

## PHYSICAL HANDICAP

### General considerations

Adaption to chronic physical disease or handicap is on the whole easier in childhood than in adult life. This is particularly so when a condition is present from birth or develops in early life and the child never knows existence without it. Even with handicaps of later onset, the plasticity of the developing personality can allow for miracles of adaption to crippling conditions. It is important that handicapped children should not be considered 'different'. They have the same human needs, physical, social and emotional, as their normal peers, and most have potentialities for developing socially useful and satisfying lives. In some, the handicap seems to motivate a heroic desire to succeed. History is full of biographies of handicapped individuals who distinguished themselves in various ways. Helen Keller, who, in spite of being both blind and deaf, made a great success of life is a good example.

### Chronic physical handicap has impact on:

*The child*—and can make him feel inadequate and inferior, particularly as he nears adolescence when the drive toward conformity with peers and rebellion against parental restrictions are usual.

*The parents* – who are often ambivalent toward him and overcompensate for their feelings of exasperation (sometimes repugnance), and guilt by undue permissiveness or giving him attention to the detriment of siblings.

*Society*. Kershaw (1961) has shown that public tolerance toward cripples varies considerably. Thus, blindness evokes great sympathy, but cerebral palsy very little, possibly because it may interfere with appearance and social habits. Obviously a child's attitudes toward himself depends upon the opinions of others around him. During middle childhood physical defects become a focus of comment and teasing, which may amount to outright cruelty. The attitudes of parents and teachers will, of course, affect the response of peers, and much can be done in

the classroom to help develop sympathetic attitudes toward less fortun-
ate individuals.

It is obvious that the total management of the physically disabled
child must involve:

● Attention to the child's *psychological response*. Dependency must be
discouraged and efforts made to establish a positive approach to the
difficulties imposed by the handicap and the development of self-reliance.

● Parents must be helped to realise that *overprotection* may result in
psychological crippling which can be more severe than the primary
physical condition. Certain risks may have to be taken but an element of
chance enters into all aspects of development, and a timid, overanxious
child is additionally handicapped. The goal must be to raise a well
adjusted child within the limits of his disability.

● Parents need practical advice on *day to day management*. There are
various voluntary organisations, for example the Diabetic and the Spina
Bifida Associations, which offer help. As the child gets older he too will
benefit from the realisation that others suffer from the same problems as
he does when he joins the group activities provided by these societies.


### Specific conditions

Obviously only some of the handicaps of childhood can be discussed.
*The epileptic child* is particularly exposed to social prejudice; since public
attitudes have not kept pace with work relating to the physiology of the
brain, and ignorance and bigotry are common. Prescription of anticonvulsant medication is only half the treatment of the epileptic. Parents
should be helped to understand that there is no disgrace in having an
epileptic child. They and the child, if old enough, must be helped toward
an understanding of what happens during a fit, and the parents of its
immediate management. They must be warned that it may be some time
before a suitable anticonvulsant regimen is found, but reassured that very
adequate control of seizures can be achieved in the vast majority of cases,
providing medication is taken regularly.

Most epileptic children can attend school normally. If there is a
chance of a major seizure occurring at school, the teacher must be advised
of the possibility and how to manage it. Restriction of activities can be
particularly irksome. There are no hard and fast rules and each case
requires individual consideration. Physical activity does not as a rule
precipitate fits and no restrictions should be placed on play with other

children in the playground. Swimming should always be under the eye of a responsible adult. The matter of bicycle riding must be decided upon the frequency and nature of the attacks and where the child rides; it is generally wise to insist that the child remains off the roads.

If handicapping attitudes and emotional and behavioural problems become apparent, these children can be helped by psychotherapy, particularly in a group situation where they can interact with other children suffering from handicapping conditions or epilepsy itself.

Several studies have indicated that *children with diabetes* have an increased incidence of emotional disturbance; attitudes of dependency, anxiety and hostility are prevalent (Shirley 1963). Acute emotional disturbance can affect diabetic control, thus, attention to the child's emotional status becomes particularly important. Most children accept the dietetic restrictions associated with the condition well, but adolescence may bring problems of denial and rebellion, and psychiatric help may be urgently needed.

*Cerebral palsy* and *spina bifida* may be associated with problems of abnormal appearance, mobility, and bladder and bowel control. Many severely affected children are catered for in centres designed specifically for them, nevertheless the aim should always be to encourage them to interact with physically normal children as much as possible.


## CHILDREN WHO HAVE ACCIDENTS

Accidents take a heavy toll of children's lives and health. Between the ages of 1 and 14 years, one half of the children who die do so as the result of an accident. As only deaths due to accidents are recorded, it is not possible to give figures for morbidity, but it is estimated that serious injuries outnumber deaths by 100 or 150 to 1. The peak incidence is at 5 years, boys outnumber girls at all ages, but the difference between sexes becomes progressively greater throughout childhood.

Whether or not 'accident prone' personalities occur is a matter of controversy, although it is self evident that an impulsive or a clumsy child will be more likely to run into difficulty than others. It is possible that a child, unable to express his aggressive impulses may unconsciously seek other ways of discharging aggression, for example by harming himself. Children who take drug overdoses and burned children very frequently came from disturbed and socially disorganised families. Parental personality, in that it affects child supervision, is an important factor in accidents involving younger children. There are often pre-existing problems before others develop as sequelae to the accident.

The management of *severely burned children* is important and challenging work. It is becoming the practice to employ a team in their care. Ward sister, surgeon, psychiatrist, physiotherapist, occupational therapist, social worker and school teacher are involved, each to a greater or lesser degree.

The psychological aspects of management involve:

● Maintaining and *improving communication* between child, staff and family.

● *Supporting* the child while he faces repeated operations and painful experiences.

● Helping the child *come to terms with his deformities*. Many are severely scarred and their appearance greatly altered. Some may be physically handicapped as the result of contractures.

● Helping the *staff in their attitudes* toward the child; in early stages he may be unpleasant to touch yet he needs physical contact and cuddling quite as much as other children.

● Making sure the child is *not bored* and unoccupied. His stay in hospital is often several months, and schooling must be arranged.

● *Planning the return home* and to school where he will have to adjust to his disfigurement in the outside world.

● Offering the *family support* and helping parents deal with the guilt they feel over the child's misfortune.

● *Preventing overprotective attitudes* on the parent's part and discouraging dependency and invalidism on the part of the child.

Research into the preventive aspects of childhood accidents is most important. There is great need to clarify what psycho-social factors predispose to accidents and how to detect children at risk.


## TERMINAL ILLNESS

This is an agonising ordeal for parents and may tax the emotional resources of medical and nursing staff to the full. When the diagnosis is certain and explanations have been given, parents should be encouraged to help in the care of their child and to spend as much time with him as possible; otherwise they may regret lost opportunities after he has gone.

Lindemann (1944) has described how families often show an anticipatory grief reaction starting to mourn before the child dies. During this process they become emotionally detached; hospital staff may react in similar fashion because they feel guilty that medical science has failed and anxious lest demands are made of them which they are unable to meet. Thus their approach to the child is impersonal and often has a superficial cheerfulness which leaves him uneasy. Hinton (1967) has shown that it is the severing of human ties and loneliness which the dying patient feels acutely rather than the threat of final dissolution. Children sense far more than adults realise; most children over about 5 years seem aware that the situation is serious and as the end approaches, become more resigned and seldom mention the future. Others adopt an attitude of denial and forced brightness, as if attempting to protect their parents from the facts. If parents cannot offer the child the personal contact he so badly needs, hospital staff should be prepared to step into their place, to show a continuing interest in the child's day to day activities and comfort, and to give him an opportunity to ask questions of an adult whom he trusts. The child's interests should be encouraged as long as possible. A daily trip to the occupational therapy department, if it can be managed, will break ward routine and offer a change of surroundings.

A major difficulty in modern hospitals is that so many staff are involved in the care of a patient, that parents feel that no one has a personal interest in their family and that there is nobody with whom they can discuss their feelings. It is essential that one person, clergyman, doctor or a member of the nursing staff be available to give support whenever it is needed and to answer questions as they arise.

The effect of a child's death upon his whole family must be considered. Siblings may feel rejected as parents spend more and more time with the dying child. Rivalry between children is normal and shouts of 'I wish you were dead', not uncommon. Given the child's belief that wishes influence events (magical thinking), it is not surprising that some brothers and sisters experience considerable guilt when a child actually dies, in addition to anxieties regarding his fate after death. Parents, and others must be prepared to answer questions about the latter.

An interview with the parents should be arranged several weeks after the death in order to discuss any worries they have regarding the nature of the illness and its treatment. Many feel guilty lest they neglected something during the child's lifetime; some may become seriously depressed and require psychiatric help.

There is no optimal way of dealing with terminal illness. Each case requires individual consideration. However, the need for one person to be closely involved and offer continuous support to the family during this tragic period cannot be over emphasised.

## CLINICAL EXAMPLES

### Chronic recurrent abdominal pain

Paul, aged 11 years was seen for consultation in a surgical ward. He had been admitted with a history of episodes of abdominal pain over 3 years. No physical basis had been found and he had no attacks while in hospital. He was an exemplary patient, quiet and conforming and helpful to nurses. His middle-aged mother regarded him as 'very precious'. She had abandoned hope of conceiving a child when she found herself pregnant with him. She said he was a 'sickly baby' but there seemed little basis for this assumption.

History taking revealed a series of family difficulties and an increasingly unhappy child. Paul's father had suffered a back injury 4 years previously and had spent a considerable time in hospital. He said he was unable to work and became increasingly morose but there was some doubt as to the underlying basis for his symptoms. His mother started a business to supplement the family income but this failed and she had to take employment outside the home. This coincided with the onset of Paul's symptoms. The family doctor was non-committal, mother was anxious for other opinions, and father felt the boy should 'pull himself together'. Paul's school work deteriorated and each time his father went into hospital his attacks became worse. Finally, he became quite morbid, talking about death and on one occasion, swallowed several aspirin tablets, as he said 'things were too bad' for him.

This family responded well to an approach which involved explaining the nature of Paul's symptoms and practical help with their very real problems. During family therapy sessions the mother was able to ventilate her resentment about being forced into the role of bread-winner. The father did eventually find work commensurate with his disability and mother was able to spend more time at home. Paul was encouraged in peer-group activities and in interests outside his home. When seen for follow-up 1 year later, there had been no more attacks of pain and Paul was functioning well both at home and at school.

### 'Invalidism' in a 12-year-old girl

Charmaine was referred with a history of three admissions to hospital for 'dizziness and fainting spells'. She had a rare congenital heart abnormality, compatible with a reasonably active life but not amenable to surgery. She had spent some time in hospital in early childhood, and was often used as a 'teaching case'. A resident noted in her chart 'this child derives considerable pleasure from having groups of students around the bed'.

Charmaine's father had been killed in an accident 3 years previously. He was replaced at the home by her mother's *de facto* husband, who strongly resented Charmaine and made no effort to hide his feelings. Charmaine was the youngest of 5 and was skilled at acting the baby in order to get others to meet her needs. She was of low-average intelligence. Because of this and frequent absences, she had fallen badly behind at school. She had been introduced to her teachers as a delicate child and was not allowed to play sport. On one occasion she exerted herself, became breathless and then discovered that over-breathing did make her feel dizzy. This was the start of her 'attacks'. She found that hyperventilation would produce faintness and on two occasions fell to the floor.

Once in hospital, Charmaine became a cheerful invalid. She described her symptoms with relish, especially to male medical students. Her three dearest wishes were to be in hospital for a long time; to have mother visit her every day and bring her chocolates and although she knew she must go home, return to hospital whenever she felt weak.

There was no doubt that this child's psychological crippling surpassed any physical handicap resultant to her cardiac condition. Arrangements were made for her admission to a convalescent home where a sympathetic, but firm approach on the part of the staff helped her realise that she could get more out of life in an active, as opposed to a passive role. She also received remedial help with school work. Social worker involvement with her family improved matters in the home to some extent, but it seems likely that interpersonal difficulties will remain.

## Diabetes in adolescence

Roger, aged 15 years, was referred with a request by his physician that he 'be locked up until he can control himself'. He was a diabetic, first diagnosed at the age of 8 and until 18 months before his visit had proved a model patient. He was the youngest of four, and the only boy. His troubles started when he began high school. His parents were ambitious and insisted that instead of going to a local school as most of his friends did, he travelled a considerable distance to a large central school 'where the teaching was better'.

Roger's mother described herself as a perfectionist. She was also the dominant partner in the marital relationship. Roger had always tended to argue with her and she 'refused to let little things go'. With the onset of puberty quarrels increased, fights developed over minor matters, then over major issues. Roger wanted more pocket money, refused to return home at times specified and became sullen and unco-operative at home. Overall his behaviour was not too atypical for this period of life, especially for a male adolescent who was probably subjected to more than his share of female dominance. Unfortunately, he started using his diabetes as a weapon. At first he would eat excessive amounts of carbohydrate, then as his relationship with his family deteriorated, started giving himself extra insulin. Finally, he was admitted to hospital in hypoglycaemic coma.

He proved a difficult patient, angry and unco-operative and responded poorly to attempts to discuss his problems with him. After many vicissitudes, a male social worker managed to establish a relationship with him and to act as intermediary between Roger and his family. Eventually, under his guidance, he was able to return home.

*Terminal illness*

Peter was diagnosed as suffering from leukaemia when he was 8. Two years later he was admitted to hospital in the final stages of the disease. His parents described their experiences as they hoped other parents in a similar position might be helped in the realisation that others had trodden the same path. They expressed themselves, sometimes hesitantly, sometimes with sudden insight over a period of several weeks as they came to grips with the situation and awaited the inevitable.

Initially, there was a forlorn hope that a cure would be found. Mother said 'I know it is wishful thinking, but while there's life there's hope. It's terrible to accept, I can't see the end, we try to live from day to day'. Peter attended the occupational therapy department daily, often in the company of his parents, and here his activities reflected this attitude of day to day living. He developed an attachment for an ancient and battered typewriter. His parents encouraged him to use it, and his increasing proficiency became a matter of great moment. This typewriter probably did more for him than anything and he died with it beside his bed.

A major concern of the parents was that they might be called upon to decide whether more treatment should be given to prolong life. This in fact did not occur, but they anticipated that it might, and needed to discuss it. Mother said, 'We'd hate to decide to continue treatment if it gave him pain. He'd be suffering for us. When it comes (the end), we want it to come quickly and hope we'll be brave enough to be with him'.

Their other concern was the extent of Peter's knowledge of his condition. He had been told there was something wrong with his blood. However, they felt that he knew more than was realised. They had always adopted the attitude that one should not lie to children, but a few weeks before when faced with Peter's question, 'Have I got the same as Aunty B, she died, didn't she ?' they panicked and said, 'No, something different', although, in fact, she had died from leukaemia. They said, 'He's listening all the time, he must put two and two together. We know he's worrying because his eyes become glazed and watery'. Father reported, 'He's always fighting to get better, if he was told he'd just throw up the sponge'. Both were very afraid that some member of the staff might, through a slip of the tongue, let Peter know the worst.

Peter's sister, aged 6 years, had been left at home with relations several miles from the hospital. She had been prepared for his death, but the parents felt acutely the difficulties in communicating with her and estimating the extent of her comprehension. She and Peter had always been very fond of each other and she showed little jealousy when they spent more and more time with Peter; they felt that they often spoiled her in their attempts to compensate for this. Subsequently she visited the hospital, although Peter was overjoyed to see her, the parents worried about her reaction to their distress. This family had a strong religious background and an experienced hospital chaplain gave them much support. Peter did not ask questions as to what would happen, but it seems unlikely that he did not know. There were times when he seemed to be making efforts toward gaiety and nonchalence. However, as time progressed, both he and his parents settled into the routine of day-to-day living described above. When the end came both parents were able to be with him.

Three months after his death, Peter's family were anxious to discuss his final days and were reassured about the extent of his suffering. Both parents had come to the realisation that a lost child is unique and cannot be replaced, but they planned realistically to continue having other children later. Their memories of him were associated with feelings of satisfaction that they had spent so much time at the hospital and were able to support him as he died. They kept and treasured his last typewriting effort, a letter addressed to them.

# BIBLIOGRAPHY

## References

*1. Psychophysiological disorders*
APLEY J. & MACKEITH R. (1968). *The Child and His Symptoms.* 2nd ed. Oxford, Blackwell Scientific Publications p. 9, p. 53, p. 57.
APLEY J. (1975). *The Child with Abdominal Pain.* 2nd ed. Oxford, Blackwell Scientific Publications.
BRITISH MEDICAL JOURNAL. (1974). *Editorial.* Normal short children, 4, 308.
BRUCH H. (1974). Eating disturbances in adolescence in *American Handbook of Psychiatry* – S. Arieti Ed-in-Chief. New York. Basic Books. Vol. II. Chapter 18.
DODGE J.A. (1976). Recurrent abdominal pain in children. *Brit. Med. J.*, 1, 385–387.
PINKERTON P. (1974). Inpatient treatment of children with psychosomatic disorders, in *The Residential Psychiatric Treatment of Children.* ed. Barker, P. London, Crosby, Lockwood Staples. p. 143.

*2. Illness and hospitalisation*
JONES P.J. (1976). Personal communication.
RICHMOND J.B. (1958). The paediatric patient in illness, in *The Psychology of Medical Practice.* ed. Hollander, M.H. Philadelphia, W.B. Saunders. Ch. 8.
ROBERTSON J. (1970). *Young Children in Hospital.* 2nd ed. London, Tavistock Publications Ltd.

*3. Chronic physical handicap*
KERSHAW J.D. (1961). *Handicapped Children.* London, Heinemann.
SHIRLEY H.F. (1963). The physically handicapped child (diabetes) in *Paediatric Psychiatry.* Massachusetts, Harvard University Press. p. 530.

*4. Terminal illness*
HINTON J. (1967). *Dying.* Ringwood, Victoria. Penguin Books Australia Ltd.
LINDEMANN E. (1944). The symptomatology and management of acute grief. *Amer. J. Psychiat.*, 101, 141–148.

## General reading

*1. Psychophysiological disorders*
APLEY J. (1975). *The Child with Abdominal Pain.* 2nd ed. Oxford, Blackwell Scientific Publications.
APLEY J. & MACKEITH R. (1968). *The Child and His Symptoms.* 2nd ed. Oxford. Blackwell Scientific Publications.
FRANK I. & POWELL M. (1967). *Psychosomatic Ailments in Childhood and Adolescence.* Springfield, Charles C. Thomas.
GARDNER L.I. (1969). Short stature associated with maternal deprivation syndrome – so called idiopathic hypopituitarism in *Endocrine and Genetic Diseases of Childhood.* ed. L.I. Gardner. Philadelphia and London, W.B. Saunders. p. 77.
PINKERTON P. (1974). *Childhood Disorders. A Psychosomatic Approach.* London, Crosby Lockwood Staples.

2. *Acute illness and hospitalisation*

BINGER C.M., ABLIN A.R., FEURSTEIN R.C., KUSHNER U.H. & ZOGER S. (1969). Childhood leukaemia. *New Eng. J. Med.* **280**, 414–418. (Relates to the management of one of the commonest causes of terminal illness in childhood).

DOUGLAS J.W. (1975). Early hospital admissions and later disturbances of behaviour and learning. *Dev. Med. and Child Neurol.* **17**, (4), 456–480.

MED. J. AUST. (1975). *Special supplement. Health Care Policy relating to Children and Their Families.* Prepared by the Association for the Welfare of Children in Hospital. Vol. **2**, No. 2.

PETRILLO M. & SANGAR S. (1972). *The Emotional Care of Hospitalised Children.* Philadelphia: Lippincott Co.

VERNON D.T.A., FOLEY J.M., SIPOWICZ R.R. & SCHULMAN J.L. (1965). *The Psychological Responses of Children to Hospitalisation and Illness.* A review of the literature. Springfield, Charles C. Thomas.

Preparing the child for hospital and occupying his time when in bed.

HARVEY S. & HALES T.A. (1972). *Play in Hospital.* London, & Faber Faber.

HEALTH COMMISSION OF NEW SOUTH WALES. (1974). (Leaflet). *Your Child in Hospital.* Sydney, D. West, Govt. Printer.

JESSEL G. in collaboration with JOLLY H. (1972). *Paul in Hospital.* London, Methuen's Children's Books.

3. *Chronic physical disease*

CROWTHER D. (1967). Psychosocial aspects of epilepsy. *Paed. Clin. of Nth. Amer.* **14**, 4, 921–33.

DRASH A. (1971). Diabetes mellitus in childhood. A review. *J. Paediat.* **78**, 6, 933.

FASSLER J. (1974). *Howie Helps Himself.* Toronto, George J. McLeod. (Shows how a boy with cerebral palsy copes with his difficulties).

MARSHALL A. (1955). *I can Jump Puddles.* London, Cheshire. (The autobiography of a cripple). Republished Australian Classic Series by Golden Press, 1974.

SHIRLEY H.F. (1963). The Physically Handicapped Child, in *Paediatric Psychiatry.* Massachusetts, Harvard University Press. Ch XIII.

4. *Accidents in childhood*

ALLAN J.L. (1976). Childhood accidents. *Aust. Paediat. J.* 12, 113–117.

BERNSTEIN, N.R., SANGER, S. & FRAS I. (1969). The functions of the child psychiatrist in the management of severely burned children. *J. Amer. Acad. Child Psychiat.* 8, 4, 620–636. (*Annual Progress Vol. 3, 1970).

KATZ J. (1976). Psychiatric aspects of accidental poisoning in childhood. *Med. J. Aust.* 2, 59–62.

VAUGHN G. (1965). Accident Proneness, in *Modern Persepctives in Child Psychiatry.* ed. Howells G.J. London, Oliver and Boyd.

*See Appendix B.

# Chapter 9
# Bad Habits. Developmental Disorders.
# Educational Problems.
# Acute and Chronic Brain Syndromes.

'Speak roughly to your little boy.
And beat him when he sneezes;
He only does it to annoy
Because he knows it teases.'

*Alice in Wonderland.*
Lewis Carroll. (Charles Lutwidge Dodgson) 1832–1898.

## 'BAD HABITS'

Persistent disturbances in patterns of sleeping or eating or excessive self-stimulation by thumb sucking, rocking or playing with genitals, not uncommonly bring parents to a clinic or family doctor's surgery. Such 'habits' do not merit a place in the classificatory system described in Chapter 3 but may of course, be associated with underlying emotional disturbance. Transient 'habits' are common enough in childhood and if any type of behaviour attracts family attention, it tends to persist; this is all the more likely if parent–child relationships are unsatisfactory.

### Sleep disturbance in the preschool child

Normally the neonate sleeps for about 20 of the 24 hours. By 1 year there is a long sleep at night and two daytime naps. By $1\frac{1}{2}$ years one of the daytime naps is dropped and usually by 3 years one long night sleep becomes sufficient. Patterns of sleep disturbance at this age include:
● *Refusal to settle.* The child demands increasingly complex rituals and inevitably this culminates in a parent lying down with him before he goes to sleep.
● Wakening during the night; sooner or later he is taken into his parents' bed.
● Wakening very early in the morning.
*These disturbances may develop because of:*
● Physical problems e.g. enlarged adenoids which give the child a feeling of suffocation when he lies down.
● Excessive sleep during the day.

● Lack of exercise e.g. the child cooped up all day in a high rise flat.

● Too much excitement before bed-time or too much noise.

● An exaggeration of the negativistic behaviour of the toddler which reaches a climax at bed-time when mother (let alone her child) is tired and fractious.

*Management.* The patience of Job in both parents and doctor is an asset. Kindly firmness is essential but often parents fear the remarks of neighbours precipitated by a screaming child, and give in to the child's demands in order to keep the peace. An experienced baby sitter will often demonstrate how well the child can settle. A night light and favourite toys in moderation are allowable but not time-consuming rituals. Establishment of an improved day time routine and attention to the parents' attitudes is more important than the use of hypnotics e.g. chloral or promethazine (see appendix A), which should only be used on a short term basis if they are used at all. Demands to come into the parents' bed during the night features in most children. However, if this is allowed to get out of hand one should question why it has happened. Does mother welcome the child's presence as a means of separating her from the father or is she so anxious about him that she craves continuous physical contact ?

## Sleep disturbances in older children

These may be classified as, 1, disorders of arousal associated with delayed C.N.S. maturation (somnambulism and night terrors) and 2, those associated with psychological disturbance (bad dreams or nightmares). *Sleepwalking* occurs in up to 6% of school children and is of little significance unless the child exposes himself to danger. *Night terrors* occur in up to 3% of children (Fenton 1975) and may persist into adult life. Typically the child emits a piercing scream and sits up in bed with staring eyes and every sign of fear. He is quite out of contact, and it is impossible to communicate with him, nor has he any memory of the event in the morning. Diazepam or nitrazepam are effective in the treatment of night terrors (Anders & Wentem 1972).

*Nightmares* or frightening dreams are often associated with overexcitement during the day. The child wakens crying and can be comforted. Both nightmares and night terrors become accentuated if the child is under stress. Neurotic children may have difficulty in settling to sleep, have terrifying dreams, or ruminate about events which have occurred during the day. Hyperkinetic and brain damaged children may sleep remarkably little, or very heavily.

Complaints of *excessive drowsiness*, especially falling asleep in class, may be related to late hours spent in front of the television set. Occasionally medication may be the culprit, for example high doses of an anticonvulsant given to an epileptic child.

### Food refusal and food fads

Studies have shown that if left to themselves young children will select an adequate diet over a period of time. However, many parents worry about the amount their children eat and try to coerce the child into routines of eating. After the first year of life the child's calorie requirements drop, and there is a considerable reduction in appetite. Since this coincides with a time when oppositional behaviour is common, the child finds food refusal a powerful way of manipulating parents. A child may refuse to eat, or eat and vomit, or eat only certain items. The author had one patient who existed for several months on avocado pears. The relationship between the gut and the emotions in childhood is very close, and the more disturbed mealtimes become, the less likely is the child to feel hungry.

*Management* should be along the following lines:

● Careful *physical examination* is mandatory. If the child is healthy and well within the norms of height and weight for his age, parents can be reassured. If he is rather thin but has no history of illness, the term 'wiry' is one in which parents find comfort.

● Sensible, easy to understand *advice about mealtimes* must be given. Small portions which are removed without comment if they are uneaten should be the rule, and no substitute offered. Refusal to allow the child to stuff himself with snacks (often biscuits) in between meals, or large amounts of milk is important.

● If a mother is unduly involved with the child's food intake, it is wise to give her time to *ventilate her anxieties*, and to help her adopt more realistic attitudes. Sometimes she may require help herself because of underlying personality difficulties.

Tonics are contraindicated.

### Pica

The eating of unnatural substances, e.g. wood, or even garden snails, is not uncommon among seriously disturbed (often emotionally deprived), mentally subnormal, or autistic children. Lead-containing paint can be ingested, with resultant chronic ill health, brain damage and mental subnormality. Management must be directed toward the underlying problems and improving the environment.

## *Auto-erotic or self-stimulating behaviour*

Thumb sucking, rocking and genital stimulation are all indulged in for a time, then discarded in favour of others interests. Children who are emotionally deprived, lack stimulation, or are intellectually handicapped, tend to persist in these habits. Rocking may be associated with head banging, which often starts in the teething period and skull fractures have occasionally been produced by a persistent knocking against cot bars or walls. Treatment must begin with an effort to discover what underlies these habits, then be directed toward the underlying cause. Parents may need reassurance that most young children show interest in their genitals, and sometimes those of their playmates. They should be advised not to draw too much attention to the habit; that punishment makes it secretive, and therefore more attractive; and to divert the child's interests into other activities.

## *Nail biting*

This is not associated with psychological disturbance, although tense, anxious children indulge more than placid ones. It reaches a peak at about 6 years, but may persist into puberty or beyond. Between 5 and 18 years, two fifths of children bite their nails. At 18 this diminishes to one third of the population (Freedman & Kaplan 1967). Treatment should be directed toward encouraging the child to take a pride in the appearance of his hands, a task more easily accomplished in girls which whom nail varnish may produce restraint. Painting bitter substances on fingers is not recommended.

## *Masturbation*

Masturbation in older children worries parents if they discover it and may engender considerable guilt in the child. In addition to solitary activity, mutual and group masturbation may occur. The youngster and his parents need reassurance that indulgence does not mean the individual is mentally abnormal. Emotionally deprived and socially isolated children, especially those in institutions where heterosexual contacts are curtailed, and inadequate individuals whose interests and activities are restricted, may masturbate excessively.


## TICS

Tics or habit spasms are defined as *sudden, involuntary, repetitive, purposeless movements of circumscribed groups of muscles.*

About 5% of children suffer from tics at some time, and the incidence reaches a peak at 7 years. Affected boys outnumber girls by 3 to 1. Tics involve the eyes, facial muscles, shoulders, vocal apparatus and feet, in descending order of frequency. The prognosis is good: at least one half recover over a 5 year period, and two thirds over 8 years. Obsessional traits in the patient, or the development of coprolalia (obscene utterances), are bad prognostic features.


### *Aetiology*

Torup's study (Corbett 1969) of 180 ticquers showed emotional disturbance associated with home or school difficulties in every case, and the general opinion is that they are exaggerated motor responses to stress. The child cannot tolerate a build up of tension and it overflows into useless motor activity. However, sometimes tics may follow disease of the central nervous system, for example encephalitis and Pasamanick has shown an association between perinatal cerebral damage and the development of tics later in life. A delay in maturation of the central nervous system has also been suggested.


### *Differential diagnosis*

A study by Apley (Apley & MacKeith 1968) showed that four fifths of children referred with a diagnosis of chorea, had tics. The differences between the two are as follows:
● Tics are more common.
● Chorea involves whole body musculature.

● The same movement is not repeated in chorea.
● Chorea is associated with hypotonia and incoordination. There is often a 'hung-up' patellar reflex.
● The E.S.R. may be raised in chorea.
In both, the movements stop during sleep.
Choreoathetoid cerebral palsy, myoclonic epilepsy and torsion spasm are occasionally confused with tics.

## Treatment

Must be directed toward stress in the background rather than the symptom itself. Parental exhortation, bribery or punishment must be discouraged since restrictions tend to aggravate the condition.

Feed-back procedures i.e. asking the child to record his movements which presumably increases awareness of the symptom, can be of value (Graham 1976). Drugs are seldom necessary, unless the child is excessively anxious.

### Gilles de la Tourette Syndrome

Here multiple tics start in childhood. Gradually barks and grunts are added and these progress to explosive, obscene utterances (coprolalia). The aetiology is unknown, but a neurological basis is suggested. Haloperiodol (Serenace) is sometimes helpful.

## HAIR PULLING (TRICHOTILLOMANIA)

This is probably not as rare as is suggested in the literature. It is commoner in girls and may be so severe as to denude a considerable area of scalp. Eyebrows and eyelashes may be removed as well. The habit does not appear to cause pain but certainly causes comment. One 8-year-old girl was called 'mothballs' by her playmates. Although superficially many of these children seem unconcerned with their appearance, the tension engendered by ridicule probably aggravates the behaviour. Generally it is regarded as an obsessional symptom (see p. 105). Most of the children come from a background in which emotional deprivation has been evident for a long period.

Several methods of treatment have been advocated, such as clipping the hair close to the scalp, wearing a wig, making arrangements to channel energy into more constructive activity, psychotherapy and family therapy (Mannito 1969). Probably a combination of occupational and family therapy offers the most hope. Unless treated early, this habit may become most persistent.

## DEVELOPMENTAL DISORDERS

Abnormalities in development associated with biological maturational lag are recognised in the following areas:
● Bladder and bowel control.
● Language and the acquisition of speech.
● Activity and attention span.
● Perceptual abilities – which affect skills such as reading.
● Motor coordination.
Although considerable variations are found in individual rates of maturation, marked delays may be evident in some children and are commoner in males and in first borns. Even though organic factors may be basic, environmental factors (especially the attitude of parents toward symptoms) influence the clinical picture and some of these disorders appear to be the result of *a maturational defect plus faulty learning because of mismanagement at a critical time.* This must be kept in mind in planning treatment.

### *Enuresis*

*Definition.* Inappropriate voiding of urine at an age when control of micturition should have been achieved. Most children are dry by day at 2–3 years and by night at 3–4 years. Wetting after 5 years is abnormal.
*Prevalence.* Complaints of enuresis, generally bedwetting, are extremely common. Although the true prevalence may be higher because parents are reluctant to complain about something 'dirty' or perhaps due to mismanagement, figures for bedwetting are generally given as:

|  |  |  |
|---|---|---|
| 5 years old | – | 10% |
| 10 years old | – | 5% |
| Teenage | – | 2% |
| Army recruits | – | 2% |

Boys come for treatment twice as commonly as girls (this may also reflect parental attitudes). The condition is commoner among the intellectually dull and those in poor social circumstances. However, it also shows a familial incidence regardless of circumstances. One third of bedwetters wet by day.

*Aetiology.* Enuresis is best regarded as a symptom which may be associated with:

● Biological maturational lag (developmental disorder).

● Faulty training.

● Emotional disturbance which results in regressive behaviour.

● Physical disease (rare).

*Patterns of enuresis.* Primary, where the child has never been dry is generally regarded as a maturation disorder affecting the neuro-muscular control of the bladder plus (often) faulty conditioning. The constitutional nature is shown by the positive family history in 70% of cases and a higher concordance rate in monozygotic as opposed to dizygotic twins. However, stress at the time of training, e.g. admission to hospital or inconsistent or punitive methods which make the child anxious, aggravate the problem. 'The bedwetting of immaturity may pass without break into the bedwetting of insecurity' (Apley & MacKeith 1968). Rarely congenital abnormalities of the urogenital system or spina bifida of sufficient degree to produce other neurological deformities may produce it, often because of associated urinary tract infections. A number of enuretic children are reported to sleep more deeply than others. Phimosis and intestinal parasites do not cause enuresis. *Secondary enuresis* which occurs after the child has been trained is practically always associated with emotional disturbance and some children wet whenever tension rises at home. In a very small number of cases there may be a physical basis, e.g. urinary tract infections, degenerative disease of the nervous system, polyuria associated with diabetes, or incontinence associated with an epileptic fit.

*Treatment.* In 1544, Phaire (Boke of Chyldren) wrote of 'Pissing in the Bedde' and suggested that ingestion of a powder made from 'the wesande of a cocke, stones of a hedgehogge or clawes of a goate' would improve matters, presumably by absorbing moisture. Penile clamps were a later innovation. Today's treatment is as follows:

● Personal involvement. The management of nocturnal enuresis is *a test of good doctoring.* An interested and energetic approach is of far more use than years of sporadic, half-hearted attempts.

● Family tension may be considerable. It is necessary to explain to parents why punitive measures should be stopped and to instil confidence as to a satisfactory outcome.

● In a private interview with the child it should be explained to him that
*he is not alone* (others suffer as well), nor is he bad, or in need of punishment. He should practise 'holding on' during the day. This serves to
increase bladder capacity and awareness of cues associated with a full
bladder. There is no need to restrict fluid intake unduly before bed. A
chart on which he inserts a silver paper star for every dry night gives him
something to show his progress.

● *Regular follow-up visits* are essential.

● If parents wish to lift the child during the night, this may be allowed
for a while, but the aim should be to stop it as soon as possible.

● *Drug treatment.* Tricyclic antidepressants produce remission, but relapses may occur. The anticholinergic effect which relaxes the musculature of the bladder wall is probably a major factor in their action but it
has also been suggested that they alter the depth of sleep and may alleviate
mood disturbance if the wetting is associated with this (Poussaint &
Ditman 1965). Children under school age should be managed by training
measures only. Imipramine is given in the following dosage:

5–8 years – 25 mg, increasing to 50 mg, at night.

8 years onwards – 50 mg, increasing to 75 mg, at night.

Mothers soon find the optimal time to give tablets which should be given
for a trial period of 6 weeks. If improvement occurs, they should be
continued for 3 months, then the dosage cautiously reduced. If a relapse
occurs, the dose should be increased again. If there is no improvement,
they should be stopped and other methods tried.

● *Conditioning.* This utilises a 'pad and buzzer' apparatus which can be
hired from surgical suppliers or clinics. The child lies on two wire gauze
sheets separated by a cotton sheet and connected to an alarm (buzzer).
As he wets the cotton sheet, this completes an electrical circuit and starts
the alarm, which wakens him so that he can visit the toilet and complete
emptying his bladder. Gradually he becomes conditioned to anticipate
events and wakens to empty his bladder before the buzzer sounds. This
apparatus should be used until the child has been completely dry for
several weeks. If relapses occur, it should be reinstated. Although the
dryness may be more slowly achieved by this method than by drugs,
relapses are said to be less likely.

*Treatment failures.* Children who are intellectually dull, from non-
supportive families or in poor social surroundings, are harder to treat.
Children in institutions present particular difficulties. Sometimes
environmental factors have to be tackled first. If, after 6 months, all
attempts to achieve dryness have failed, it is wisest to explain to the

parents that the child's bladder is not yet mature enough to train, give them a rest, and then start again.

*Who treats enuresis?* Some local authorities run special clinics. Aside from these, undoubtedly the family doctor is in the best position to adopt a total approach to the child and his family. Referral for a psychiatric opinion should only be made if the wetting is associated with emotional disturbance.

## Encopresis

*Definition.* Passage of stool in an inappropriate place after the age of 3 to 4 years in the absence of any relevant organic defect. Most children achieve bowel control soon after the age of 2 years.

*Prevalence* is hard to ascertain as it is one of the least acceptable symptoms in childhood, and some parents are too ashamed to complain. Bellman (1966) reports that $1\frac{1}{2}\%$ of children are encopretic at the age of 7 to 8 years, and that boys outnumber girls by 3 to 1. The condition does not persist into adult life. It may sometimes be associated with enuresis.

*Classification.* Although there is probably a basic maturational lag which makes bowel control difficult to achieve, other factors may contribute. Three types are distinguished:

● *Primary, or 'continuous'* when the child has never achieved control. This is often associated with intellectual dullness plus inconsistent management on the part of the mother.

● *'Stress soiling'* in anxious children—an increase in family tension or exams at school are followed by episodes of encopresis. These children do not become constipated.

● *Soiling with retention.* These children are toilet trained initially but start to 'hang on' to their faeces and pass them in inappropriate places. Sometimes the child is so absorbed in play he 'forgets to go' or he dislikes using school toilets and events overtake him on the way home. Occasionally an anal fissure at the outset conditions the child to associate defaecation with pain. Anthony (1968) describes the contribution of early training. A disturbance in the relationship between 'the potting couple' – that is mother and the child she is trying to train – may result in a toddler deliberately withholding faeces in an effort to exert his authority. This is likely to happen if the mother attempts to train her child before he is physiologically ready or if he is punished excessively for soiling and becomes angry and confused. Children in this group may become severely constipated with consequent gross distension of the large bowel with hard, impacted faeces (psychogenic megacolon). Sooner or later this produces leakage of liquid faecal matter (retention with overflow or 'spurious incontinence'). The unpleasantness of the symptom often engenders punitive attitudes in parents and the child becomes angry and rebellious in his turn. By the time he reaches the doctor, the disturbance is compounded of *disturbed bowel physiology*, possibly aggravated by excessive use of laxatives and suppositories, *and a disturbed psyche*. The whole situation has become so unpleasant that the child represses cues associated with the need to defaecate.

A rare congenital condition in which nerve ganglia are absent from a segment of the colonic wall (Hirschsprungs disease) may occasionally be confused with encopresis. It is characterised by a history of constipation dating from birth, failure to thrive and the infrequent passage of large stools.

*Management.* The encopretic child is an unpopular patient, initiating feelings of repulsion in both parents and physicians, but he can be cured with time and patience. The history and examination will suggest the group to which the child belongs. Treatment will vary according to the factors involved, but essentially one must treat the whole child, 'not just the hole in him' (Pinkerton 1965). In group one, the mother should be helped to adopt correct training methods. In group two, attention must be paid to reducing anxiety and helping the child cope with stress. These children may respond to tricyclic antidepressants in the same way as those with enuresis. In group three the aims should be:

● To restore normal bowel function.
● To improve parental attitudes and management.
● To relieve the child's hostility.

It must be explained to the parents that bowel rhythm must be re-established and that this can only be achieved slowly. If the child is constipated, attention to diet and a laxative at night, together with regular 'sitting out' in the morning, is indicated. Parents must be helped to realise that punitive attitudes aggravate matters. Suppositories, which the child inevitably regards as punishment, should be stopped. Sometimes the lower colon and rectum are so overloaded that clearance by enema is an essential prelude to bowel training. If this is the case, manual disimpaction and irrigation under a general anaesthetic may be necessary to avoid further psychological trauma.

Play therapy, which allows the child to ventilate his anger and realise that he has an ally in the therapist who is interested in his progress and who encourages him toward mature behaviour and in creative activities, must go hand in hand with physical methods. Sometimes admission to a hospital psychiatric unit is advisable.

*Disorders of speech and language*

The rate of language acquisition varies considerably among normal children and in general *comprehension of speech precedes expression.* Girls are often ahead of boys; a socially stimulating environment will encourage speech development, a multilingual background does not retard it providing the child is of normal intellectual ability. Parents estimates of the extent of a child's vocabulary are often unduly optimistic since they learn to interpret incomplete expressions.

The following table 9.1 gives an outline of normal speech development:

| Age | Stage |
| --- | --- |
| 4 months | Babbling starts. This increases when the baby is spoken to, or is pleased. |
| 6 months | Vocalises deliberately as a means of interpersonal communication. Syllables such as 'dad-dad' appear, at first used indiscriminately and later are attached to specific adults. |
| 15 months | The child makes his wants known by gesture with an occasional recognisable word. Vocabulary is under 10 words, but he understands many more. |
| 2 years | Vocabulary is now 50 or more words. Puts 2 or more words together to form simple sentences. |
| 2½ years | Vocabulary over 200 words. Continually asks questions. |
| 3 years | Now has a large vocabulary. Talks to himself in monologues. Able to verbalise past experience and to take part in conversation. |
| 4 years | Speech is clear with a few infantile vocalisations. The child gives a comprehensive account of himself and tells stories. |

*Pathology.* It is important to distinguish between language disorders which involve the use and comprehension of words, and disorders which involve the motor aspects of speech. *Speech disorders* include:

● Defects of voice, e.g. due to paralysis of the laryngeal muscles or to functional disorder in older children, when a hoarse whisper is generally produced.
● Dysarthria or disorders of articulation, which are associated with physical defects in tongue, palate, nerves or muscles associated in speech.
● Developmental problems where an infantile form of speech persists (dyslalia).
● Dysrhythmias – stammering or stuttering.
● Secondary disorders relating to underlying problems such as mental retardation or deafness.

A tendency to stammer may develop at about 4 or 5 years, a period of particularly rapid speech development. In some cases it may persist;

although parental anxiety and mismanagement may contribute to this, a basic maturational problem has been suggested.

Early treatment by a speech therapist is important. This is based on relaxation, reduction of anxiety, improving self-confidence; and parent counselling.

*Language disorders.* Sometimes the child comprehends what is said, but is unable to express himself (expressive dysphasia); if, however, he fails to comprehend (receptive dysphasia), then he will not learn to use words. Congenital dysphasia or specific language disability is thought to be associated with developmental abnormality in the central nervous system, but there may be a history suggestive of brain damage early in life. Many dysphasic children are left handed and there may be a family history of language problems. The condition varies in severity. Some children, although slow to develop language, eventually communicate quite well. In others, the handicap is severe and persistent.

Children with severe language problems are recognized by their failure to comprehend the spoken word, although they will respond to gesture, and by the production of unintelligible jargon when they should be starting to speak. Many of these children become frustrated by their failure and secondary emotional disturbance is not uncommon. Childhood autism, which has as one of its cardinal symptoms a failure in language development, is described in Chapter 10. Delayed language development may be secondary to some other factor, for example deafness, intellectual handicap, or severe socio-cultural deprivation. Twins are often slow with speech and may develop a private means of communication. '*Elective mutism*' is a term which is used rather freely and sometimes erroneously. It must be kept for children who have proven their ability to speak but elect not to do so in certain situations. Sometimes a child with a specific language disability is subjected to unjustified pressure as he is regarded as not wanting to speak rather than being unable to do so.

*Examination of the non-speaking child.* If a child has not acquired speech by $2\frac{1}{2}$ to 3 years, he should be carefully assessed. This will include:
● History taking, especially with regard to development of early vocalisation and the family history of speech development.
● Recording what speech has developed.
● Neurological examination.
● Audiometry to exclude hearing problems.
● Intellectual assessment.

Children with an established speech or language problem should be referred to a speech therapist.

*Hyperactivity/hyperkinetic syndrome/attention deficit disorder*

The hyperactive child is characterised by persistent, purposeless motor activity, a limited attention span, distractability, impulsiveness and emotional instability. The disorder may persist well into the school years and often places a severe strain upon parental tolerance and the family generally. Recognition of the severely hyperactive child is not difficult (he can wreck the doctor's office), but a mildly affected child may sit quietly in a one-to-one situation with an adult, whereas his behaviour will deteriorate quickly with a group of noisy children. The decision as to whether a child is hyperactive is a subjective one, and the term is often used loosely and imprecisely. There can be few difficult children who have not been labelled hyperactive at some stage of their lives. Parental tolerance may vary considerably, but if a child's behaviour is such that it causes *comment both in the home and outside it*, it is fair to regard it as abnormal.

Hyperactivity is thought to be associated with a C.N.S. maturational delay. A similar behaviour pattern is shown by some children known to have suffered brain damage, and it may be associated with mental subnormality or autism. Emotionally disturbed, highly anxious children are often very restless, but the pattern is less consistent than in the condition described above, nor has it the same 'driven' quality about it.

Understandably, hyperactive children produce negative reactions in their parents, but restrictions and punishment aggravate the situation. Management should be along the following lines:

● A decision must be made as to whether the parents' *complaints are justified* or whether they need help in coping with the normal exuberance of childhood.

● If behaviour can justifiably be regarded as abnormal, then the aim must be to reduce the demands made on the child to a level with which he can cope. Parents require simple explanations and reassurance that he is neither deliberately wicked nor rebellious, but is suffering from a treatable condition. It is neither his fault nor theirs. The *environment should be structured* so that he is neither overstimulated nor unduly restricted. He needs a regular, quiet routine. This can be difficult to achieve in a modern home, but much can be done to institute confident and consistent management on the parents' part if they are supported by their doctor.

● *Drugs* have an important part to play, but sometimes a trial period may be necessary to determine which is most effective. One drug must be given at a time, in adequate doses, and its effect should be assessed for several weeks. The following are used:

Psychic stimulants – These are regarded as the drugs of choice by several authorities (Barkley 1977). Methylphenidate (Ritalin) is reported to be the most effective. The dose is 5–20 mg/day but some authorities recommend much larger amounts, e.g. 80–100 mg/day (Shader 1975). Dextroamphetamine (Dexedrine) is also used. These drugs should be given early in the day to avoid sleep disturbance. With larger doses, height and weight may be affected and should be monitored. It is usual to omit the tablets during summer holidays so as to give the child a chance to catch up, and to assess the need to continue medication. Although there is no evidence that children on these potentially addictive drugs become drug dependent in later life, it is wise to restrict their use to children under 10 years. These are restricted drugs and in some States their prescriptions require endorsement.

Antipsychotic drugs, e.g. Chlorpromazine (Largactil) and thioridazine (Melleril) will quieten very restless children. They may however, impair learning. For dosage see Appendix A.

Tricyclic antidepressants have been reported to be of value in some cases. Magnesium pemoline has also been recommended but has not yet been used extensively.

Antihistamines, anticonvulsants and minor tranquillisers, e.g. diazepam have not proved effective.

Epileptic children showing hyperactivity may require the addition of methylphenidate or a tranquilliser to their anticonvulsant regimen.

There is as yet no scientific evidence that a diet which excludes salicylate derivatives and preservatives (Feingold diet) is effective (Werry 1976). It is regarded as *sub judice* at present.

Phenobarbitone should not be given to hyperactive children, as it may aggravate rather than improve the condition.

The hyperactive child may tax the patience of all in contact with him. Supportive care by the doctor, combined with the judicious use of drugs, will produce considerable improvement in most cases. Remission generally occurs as the child matures.


### *Perceptual handicap. Specific learning problems*

Although of normal intelligence and exposed to adequate teaching, some children fail to progress in specific areas of school work, commonly reading. Receptors and neuronal sensory pathways are intact, but they fail to integrate, recognise and respond appropriately to stimuli, i.e. have perceptual difficulties. Children with auditory perceptual defects show an inability or slowness to attach meanings to words, and when shown written symbols, they are unable to recall the sound equivalent. They confuse instructions, and are often labelled disobedient. Visual perceptual defects make it difficult to recognise and reproduce letters. These are often written in reverse or upside down, e.g. 'b' for 'd', 'w' for 'm'. Sometimes whole syllables may be reversed, e.g. 'god' for 'dog'. Occasionally pages of these reversals (mirror writing) may be produced. Many of these children have difficulty in integrating total sensory input, which includes tactile and kinaesthetic as well as visual and auditory cues. They may have trouble in orienting themselves in space, in relating cause to effect, and their responses to others in their environment (social perception) may be distorted.

### Abnormalities in motor development. Clumsiness

Delay in acquiring motor skills (developmental dyspraxia) can be a considerable handicap. Gross motor co-ordination, such as is involved in running or skipping, or fine motor movements and eye–hand co-ordination may be affected. Sport presents especial problems, since companions refuse to play with a child who cannot catch a ball. Writing and drawing may be extremely poor and the motor side of speech may be affected, making communication difficult. Labels such as 'stupid' or lazy are often applied and secondary emotional disturbance may bring affected individuals to attention.

### Minimal brain dysfunction

The concept of a syndrome of cerebral dysfunction manifest in behavioural and neurological dimensions was put forward by Goldstein in 1936 and extended by Strauss and Werner in 1946. Since then there has been increasing recognition that many children who present with behavioural or learning problems, suffer from irregularities in development of the central nervous system. '*Minimal brain dysfunction*' (MBD), '*minimal chronic brain syndrome*', '*minimal brain damage*' and '*attention deficit disorder*' have all been used to describe this syndrome. The first term is generally preferred as it is less disturbing for parents, and firm evidence of brain damage cannot be demonstrated in all cases. Hyperkinesis, perceptual defects which, in many cases, are associated with learning problems, language disorders and motor dysfunction, all described above, are involved. M.B.D. children are not mentally retarded and may be of average or above average intelligence. Each child presents with *an individual profile of disabilities*, some suffering from several, some from only one. Each deficit varies in degree, thus the overall picture is of a rather heterogeneous group.

*Prevalence.* Between 5–10% of school age children show evidence of M.B.D. (Wender 1971). Boys are more commonly affected than girls (probably about 6–10 to 1), as are first borns and children from poor socio-economic backgrounds.

*Aetiology.* Cerebral damage in early life, especially the perinatal period, has repeatedly been implicated but is hard to prove. Knobloch and Pasamanick (1959) refer to a continuum of reproductive casualty; at one end is the child with severe cerebral palsy, mental defect or epilepsy, at the other the child with M.B.D., with minor motor problems, perceptual difficulties, hyperactivity and minor E.E.G. abnormalities. Clustering of cases within families may occur, suggesting a genetic basis in some cases. Lopez (1965) evaluated 10 pairs of twins. The 4 monozygotic pairs were concordant for M.B.D. and 5 out of 6 dizygotic pairs were discordant. Studies of monkeys subjected to hypoxia at birth (Sechzer *et al.* 1973) showed long term sequelae and these included hyperactivity, clumsiness, defects in sensory responsiveness and meagre vocalisation. Post mortem examination showed neuronal damage associated with asphyxia, in the brain stem and diencephalon. Animals sacrificed later in life showed that neuronal deficits had escalated rather than the reverse, although this did not correlate with an increase in symptoms.

*History.* It must be remembered that each child shows an individual clinical profile, but characteristics typical of different stages of development are given below:

Infancy — The child is restless, colicky, overalert, cries excessively and said to be 'different' from siblings.

Toddler stage — Hyperactivity makes him a constant threat to himself and family possessions. He is distractable, impulsive, has a low frustration tolerance, and this produces severe frequent and temper tantrums.

Kindergarten — Now he is unpopular because of his emotional displays and aggression. His teacher calls him immature and sometimes remarks on his clumsiness. Hyperactivity

|          |                                                                      |
|----------|----------------------------------------------------------------------|
|          | may present many difficulties as physical strength increases.        |
| School   | – Clumsiness, learning problems (often not appreciated until grades 2 or 3) and emotional disturbance, are noted. Attitudes of clowning may be adopted to bolster self esteem. The child is called a nuisance, stupid or accident prone. |
| Adolescence | – Learning problems may persist or escalate, although the child may now appear hypoactive. Sociopathic behaviour may develop secondary to his frustration and social perceptual difficulties. School drop out and/or delinquency may occur. |

*Examination of the child with M.B.D.*

● General appearance. Many children show *minor anatomical abnormalities*. Sometimes they are unkindly and unscientifically referred to as 'funny looking kids'.

● Conventional neurological examination may elicit *'soft' signs*, so called because of their variability and lack of correlation with anatomical lesions. Hypertonicity in an isolated group of muscles, and an extensor plantar reflex on one side only, are common findings.

● Gross motor skills should be assessed by watching the child running, skipping and tandem walking (heel–toe) along a line.

● Fine motor movement and eye–hand co-ordination can be tested by asking the child to tie a knot, do up buttons or to write.

● When standing with hands outstretched, many of these children show a gradual drift of one arm downwards and *minor jerky (choreo-athetoid) movements*. Mirror movements are also common, for example when brushing his hair with his right hand, the child may involuntarily perform similar movements with the left.

● Perceptual function may be tested by asking the child to copy geometrical figures (see figure 9.1).

● Language function can be evaluated by the ability to follow verbal instructions and to use speech.

● Reading skills can be checked using a book appropriate to age and intellectual level.

● Many of these children show evidence of *crossed laterality* (mixed cerebral dominance). Lateral dominance may be tested by determining whether preference is shown for the right or the left hand, eye and foot. Hand preference may be tested by asking the child to write or throw a ball. Eye dominance is tested by giving the child a toy telescope or a sheet of paper with a hole in the centre, so that he can hold it and peek at the examiner through the hole. Kicking a ball is the best test of foot preference, but several trials of hopping on one foot may be used instead. The significance of inconsistent dominance is not known.

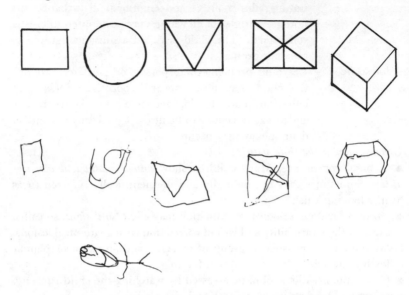

Figure 9.1. Copies of geometric figures, shown above, produced by a 10-year-old boy with M.B.D. He was of borderline intelligence and had severe visual perceptual and dyspraxic difficulties. His fine motor coordination was so poor that when copying these figures he attempted to steady his right hand, which held the pencil, with his left hand. His reading age was approximately that of a 6-year-old and his spelling age congruent. His achievement in maths was rather better. He showed left-right confusion and had considerable difficulty in orienting objects in space. When asked to draw a man (lowest line) he rotated the figure through 90°, but insisted he was standing up. His language skills were adequate. He was impulsive and distractible and presented a management problem to his elderly adoptive parents. His birth and early history were unknown, but his mother was reported to be 'not mentally normal'.

● E.E.G. recordings. Between 50–60% of children with behaviour disorders have abnormal E.E.G.'s compared with the incidence of 10–15% in normal children. Generally this consists of an excess of slow activity, which may be diffuse and characteristic of an 'immature' record, or confined to the temporal regions (Kiloh 1972).

*Psychological assessment* may demonstrate other deficits.

● Although his I.Q. is within the normal range, the child's *intellectual level is often lower than might be expected*, considering the intelligence of parents and siblings.

● On the W.I.S.C. or the W.P.P.S.I. the *verbal I.Q. is commonly 20 points or more above the performance I.Q.* However, in the presence of severe language disability, or if the child comes from an unstimulating background, the performance I.Q. may be above the verbal.

● There is often a *scatter in the subtests* of the W.I.S.C. Those involving abstraction of information are done particularly badly, for example block design or coding.

Visual perceptual difficulties may be shown on the Bender-Gestalt or Beery-Buktenica tests, and auditory perceptual difficulties on the Wepman test. Educational assessment is of great practical importance since many of these children need help in the classroom (see Chapter 5).

The psychologist may also note the child's *limited attention span and distractability.* Sometimes the child may give up in panic when confronted with a task at which he seems likely to fail ('catastrophic' reaction).

*Management.* The management of hyperactivity has already been discussed. The nature of the child's handicaps must be explained to the parents and special educational programmes arranged. Avoidance of criticism or punishment are cardinal principles. Any skills which the child has should be encouraged in an effort to boost his self-confidence.

*Prognosis.* Generally symptoms improve as the child matures. Hyperactivity diminishes and may be replaced by hypoactive behaviour. Clumsiness and learning problems tend to improve; however if present in severe degree, may persist. Menkes (1967) re-evaluated 11 cases diagnosed as suffering from M.B.D. 25 years previously and showed that 4 were psychotic, 2 mentally subnormal, and only 5 were self-supporting and of these, 4 had been institutionalised at some time; 8 had evidence of neurological impairment, and 2 remained hyperactive beyond 25 years of age. Other studies have attempted to link minimal brain dysfunction in childhood with adult psychiatric disorder. Stone (1968) suggests that patients diagnosed as suffering from simple schizophrenia may be M.B.D. children grown up, and Anderson and Plymate (1960) that even in the more benign cases, social and interpersonal difficulties persist. Perhaps the label 'minimal' is inappropriate.

*Summary.* Approximately 5–10% of the child population show behavioural and/or learning problems which are thought to be associated with dysfunction of the central nervous system. Clinical experience and animal experiments suggest that cerebral insult may be an aetiological factor, but clustering of cases in families suggest that genetic factors are involved as well. Whatever the primary condition, environmental factors, especially parental attitudes towards the handicaps, will influence the final picture. In general, hyperactivity predominates early in childhood and school problems later on. Many symptoms improve with maturation, but this is by no means always so, and it has been suggested that these children are predisposed to social failure and psychiatric illness in adult life. Treatment involves early recognition, environmental manipulation to reduce stress on the child, and teachers and parents must be helped to accept the disabilities from which the child suffers. When hyperactivity is marked, medication, often on a long-term basis, may be necessary.


## EDUCATIONAL PROBLEMS

### *General difficulty with school work*

Children may fall behind at school because of:

● *Intellectual handicap.* Milder degrees of defect may be missed until school begins. Children who function within the 60–80 I.Q. range need to go at a slower pace than their peers. Personality and motivational factors are important and individual assessment is necessary before transfer to a special school. Children below this level are capable of doing only very limited school work, and may not be educable.

● *Physical defects.* Visual defects, deafness or chronic physical illness which entails missing a considerable amount of school, will cause the child to fall behind.

● The limited attention span, distractability and impulsivity associated with *developmental hyperactivity.* This not only impairs learning, but also predisposes to social rejection.

● *Socio-cultural factors.* Difficulties are compounded of a lack of stimulation, motivation to succeed and sometimes frequent absences or changes of school.

● *Emotional factors.* Excessive anxiety not only impedes learning but may cause the child to evade situations where he has to compete with others or is exposed to criticism. Anger and hostility may be shown through negative attitudes to school work. Depression produces apathy and a poor self image and the child feels it is not worthwhile trying to achieve anything.

Obviously, the quality of teaching to which the child is exposed is important, particularly so in the case of the less gifted child. Some children present as *late maturers*; probably this is the result of minor biological developmental delays combined with social and emotional factors; individual help will often improve the negative attitudes which many develop toward school work.

## Specific learning problems

Children of average intelligence or above, may fail to progress in a particular subject, of which reading is the commonest. It has been reported that in Western society as many as 10–20% of school children suffer from reading problems. The lower rates in some countries e.g. Japan, have been explained on philological grounds. When obvious deficiencies such as inadequate teaching have been allowed for, it appears that poor readers fall into two groups (Rutter & Yule 1975), called by these authors:

- General reading backwardness.
- Specific reading retardation.

*General reading backwardness* affects boys and girls equally and these children may have additional learning problems. Overt neurological disorder and/or developmental deficits such as poor motor coordination, language and speed disorders, perceptual difficulties and left–right confusion are common among them. These children are generally from large families and lower socio-economic classes, i.e. there is a compounding of neurological and social factors.

*Specific reading retardation* is three times as common in boys (see figure 9.2) as in girls, is rarely associated with other neurological deficits, and has a familial incidence. These children are good at other school skills, for example mathematics, but have an increased incidence of language problems compared with a normal control group.

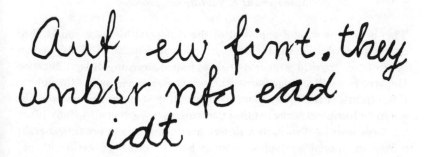

Figure 9.2. This sentence was written by a 10 year old boy who suffered from specific reading retardation. Its meaning was, he said: 'Off we went. We ran (runned) to fetch it.'

A confusing nomenclature has grown up around reading disability; 'dyslexia', 'word blindness' and 'specific reading disability' are all terms which have been used. It is probably best to apply the term *reading retardation* to children who are two years or more behind their mental age in reading and regard it as a symptom which may be related to one or several factors. These include:

● Poor teaching.
● Socio-cultural deprivation.
● Emotional problems.
● M.B.D., associated with perceptual difficulties.
● A specific defect in language development (specific reading disability).

### *The relationship between reading retardation and antisocial behaviour*

This association is generally recognised, for example Bakwin and Bakwin (1972) report a New York study of youthful law breakers which showed that 76% were 2 years or over retarded in reading. Rutter *et al.* (1975) describe common factors (parental personality problems, impoverished circumstances and an unsatisfactory school environment) which underlie both reading retardation and conduct disorders. This does not preclude some children becoming delinquent as a maladaptive response to a specific reading handicap.

### *Management of educational problems*

This involves a careful appraisal of the child and his background. The doctor's contribution will include correction of visual and auditory defects or any other physical problems likely to impede learning. State Education Departments will arrange for psychological assessment and in the light of this, reconsider the child's placement within the educational system. The guiding principle must be to tailor the school programme to the individual. Children who need to go at a slower pace than their peers are generally moved to 'special' or 'opportunity' schools. Formal education is continued, but the emphasis is on social training and the development of practical skills. Classes are small and the child receives much individual help. Children with specific learning problems are kept in the classroom doing standard work as much as possible, but allowed to attend remedial classes at certain times during the day. This reduces the chances of them coming to feel 'different' or abnormal.

## ACUTE BRAIN SYNDROMES

Delirious or confusional states associated with diffuse impairment of brain tissue function and which are temporary and reversible, occur quite commonly in association with acute infections or drug intoxication in childhood. Perhaps this is because the blood brain barrier is immature, and does not protect the brain from circulating toxins as well as it does in adults. Such conditions may last from a few hours to several days.

### Clinical features

The symptoms fluctuate in severity and are often worse at night:
● There is *clouding of consciousness* with diminished or accentuated response to stimuli.
● *Anxiety* and restlessness are prominent.
● The child is *disoriented* and only dimly aware of time of day and the identity of the people around him.
*Illusions* and *hallucinations* are common. The latter are usually visual and may be frightening.

When clouding of consciousness is of such marked degree that the patient can only be roused temporarily, he is said to be in a state of stupor. When consciousness is lost and there is no voluntary activity, in coma.

### Treatment

This is as follows:
● Identify and treat the *aetiological factors*. Counteract dehydration if necessary. Electrolyte control may be necessary.
● *Nurse in a quiet room* with constant lighting of moderate intensity throwing a minimum of shadows. Protection of the restless child is important. If mother can sit with him, so much the better.
● *Medication* to reduce restlessness may be necessary if this is severe but should not become a substitute for good nursing. Suitable preparations are chloral syrup, 2.5–5 ml by mouth; chlorpromazine, 10–25 mg depending on the age of the child, by mouth or intramuscularly; diazepam, 2–10 mg depending on the age of the child, by mouth, intramuscularly or intravenously.

## CHRONIC BRAIN SYNDROMES

These result from permanent impairment of cerebral function, associated with brain damage. They may be produced by severe infections, intoxications, degenerative disease of the brain or space occupying lesions within the skull. However, the commonest cause is head injury, often as the result of a traffic accident.

*Clinical features*

These depend upon the location and extent of the lesion, the child's reaction to his injury, and the parents' reactions and management. The following may occur:
- *Mental subnormality* of varying degree (global cognitive impairment).
- Impairment of *particular intellectual functions*, such as memory and perception.
- *Limited attention span* and distractability. The child reacts indiscriminately to stimului, and not to a situation as a whole. He may be perseverative, returning to the same task again and again. If faced with many competing stimuli, he may exhibit a 'catastrophic' reaction, losing control over his motor behaviour and emotions.
- *Hyperkinesis* (persistent purposeless motor activity) may make the child a considerable management problem.
- *Emotional lability* (tears one moment, smiles the next).
- *Focal defects* e.g. loss of speech.
- *Epileptic fits*.
Following quite severe head injury, many children make surprisingly good recovery in intellectual function and focal defects. Restlessness may improve with maturation, but disinhibited behaviour may be persistent and severe, and mitigate against satisfactory adjustment.

*Examination should include:*

- Neurological and psychological assessment.
- Family assessment. Can the parents manage a potentially difficult child, offer control without being punitive, are their expectations realistic?

## Management

● *The family need help* in accepting their child's limitations and often with their guilt about why the accident occurred. The environment should be structured so that not too many demands are made upon the child; over-stimulation should be avoided.

● Appropriate placement in the *educational system* is essential.

● *Drug treatment.* Tranquillisers, e.g. chlorpromazine or thioridazine can be of value. Long-term administration of these may be necessary, but they should be stopped from time to time to assess their continuing value. In some cases, psychic stimulants, such as amphetamine or methylphenidate may prove more effective. Anticonvulsants may be necessary to control seizures. Phenobarbitone may aggravate rather than improve behavioural difficulties.

## BIBLIOGRAPHY

### References

ANDERS T.F. & WEINSTEIN P. (1972). Sleep and its disorders in infants and children. A review. *J. Paediat.* **50**, 311–324 (*Annual Progress* Vol. 6, 1973).

ANDERSON C. & PLYMATE H.B. (1960). Managment of the brain damaged adolescent. *Am. J. Orthopsychiatry*, **32**, 492–500.

ANTHONY E.J. (1957). An experimental approach to the psychopathology of childhood: encopresis. *Brit. J. Medical Psychology*, **30**, 146–175.

APLEY J. & MACKEITH R. (1968). *The Child and His Symptoms*, 2nd ed. Oxford: Blackwell Scientific Publications. p. 125.

BAKWIN H. & BAKWIN R.M. (1972). *Behaviour Disorders in Children.* Philadelphia & London, W.B. Saunders Co. p. 575.

BARKLEY R.A. (1977). A review of stimulant drug research with hyperactive children. *J. Child Psychol. & Psychiat.* **18**, 137–65.

BELLMAN M. (1966). Studies in encopresis. *Acta Paediat. Scand.* Supp. 170.

CORBETT J.A. (1969). Tics and Giles de la Tourette Syndrome. *Brit. J. Psychiat.* **115**, 1229–1241.

FENTON G.W. (1975). Clinical disorders of sleep. *Brit. J. Hosp. Med.* **14**(2), 120–145.

FREEDMAN A.M. & KAPLAN H.I. (eds) (1967). *Comprehensive Textbook of Psychiatry.* Baltimore, Williams & Wilkins Co. p. 1383.

GRAHAM P. (1976). Management in child psychiatry, recent trends. *Brit. J. Psychiat.* **129**, 97–108.

KILOH L.G., McCOMAS A.J. & OSSELTON J.W. (1972). *Clinical Electroencephalography.* 3rd ed. London, Butterworths. p. 170.

KNOBLOCH H. PASAMANICK B. (1959). Syndrome of minimal cerebral damage in infancy. *J. Am. Med. Ass.* **170**, 1384.

LOPEZ R.E. (1965). Hyperactivity in twins. *Canad. Psychiat. Ass. J.* **10**, 421.

MANNITO F.V. & DELGADO R.A. (1969). Trichotillomania in children. *Amer. J. Psychiat.* **126**, 505–511.

MENKES M. (1967). A 25 year follow-up study on the hyperactive child with minimal brain dysfunction. *Paediatrics*, **39**, 393–399.

PINKERTON P. (1965). The psychosomatic approach in child psychiatry in *Modern Perspectives in Child Psychiatry.* ed. J.G. Howells. London, Oliver & Boyd. p. 323.

POUSSAINT A.F. & DITMAN K.S. (1965). A controlled study of imipramine in the treatment of childhood enuresis. *J. Paediat.* **67**, 283–290.

RUTTER M. YULE W. (1975). The concept of specific reading retardation. *Jnl. Child Psychol. and Psychiat.* **16**, 181–197.

RUTTER M., YULE B., QUINTON D., ROWLANDS O., YULE W. & BERGER M. (1975). Attainment and adjustment in two geographical areas. *Brit. J. Psychiat.* **126**, 520–533.

SECHZER J.A., FARO M.D. & WINDLE W.F. (1973). Studies of monkeys asphyxiated at birth: implications for minimal brain dysfunction. *Seminars in Psychiatry*, **5** (1), 19/34. (*Annual Progress* Vol **7**, 1974).

SHADER R.I. ed. (1975). *Manual of Psychiatric Therapies.* Boston, Little Brown & Co. p. 167.

STONE A., HOPKINS R. & MAHNKE M. (1968). Simple schizophrenia: syndrome or shibboleth? *Am. J. Psychiat.* 125, 305–312.

WENDER P.H. (1971). *Minimal Brain Dysfunction in Children.* New York, Wiley

WERRY J. (1976). Food additives and hyperactivity. Guest Editorial. *Med. J. Aust.* 2, 281–282.

## General reading

KOLVIN I., MACKEITH R.C. & MEADOWS R. (1973). *Bladder Control and Enuresis.* London, Spastics International Medical Publications in association with Heinemann.

PAINE R.S. & OPPE T.E. (1966). *The Neurological Examination of Children.* London, Spastics International Medical Publications in association with Heinemann. Vol 20/21. Chapters 6 & 7.

POND D. (1965). The neuropsychiatry of childhood. 1. The brain damaged child, in *Modern Perspectives in Child Psychiatry,* ed. J.G. Howells. London & Edinburgh, Oliver & Boyd.

WENDER P.H. & EISENBERG L. (1974). Minimal brain dysfunction in children. In *American Handbook of Psychiatry.* Editor-in-Chief S. Arieti. New York, Basic Books Inc. Chapter 8.

WERRY J.S. (1972). Organic factors in childhood psychopathology in *Psychopathological Disorders in Childhood*, eds. H.C. Quay, J.S. Werry. London, Wiley.

*See Appendix B.

# Chapter 10
# Psychosis in Childhood

'Curiouser and curiouser', cried Alice.

Lewis Carroll (Charles Lutwidge Dodgson) 1832–1898
*Alice in Wonderland.*

In the psychiatry of adults, psychosis signifies severe mental illness in which there is disturbed contact with reality. Psychotic children show *severely disturbed, bizarre and unpredictable behaviour*. It is thought that this results from disturbed contact with reality and that their distorted perception leads them to attach meanings to objects and events which an observer cannot comprehend and is therefore puzzled by their behaviour. Many psychotic children show mood disturbance and most, regressive behaviour, often to the extent that they are regarded as being primarily mentally retarded.

## CLASSIFICATION

Broadly these conditions fall into two groups: (1) those associated with a known disturbance in brain tissue function, and (2) those in which there appears to be no underlying physical factor and therefore are labelled functional. Failure to demonstrate neurological disorder does not mean an organic basis is necessarily absent and may not be found in the future.

### Acute toxic psychosis

Transient disturbances in brain tissue function associated with drug overdose or idiosyncrasy, or acute infections produce disturbed contact with reality see p. 173.

### Psychoses associated with chronic organic pathology

Cerebral degenerations, e.g. the lipoidoses in which fatty substances are deposited in the brain as the result of a metabolic disorder, can produce clinical pictures comparable to the other psychoses of childhood. Sometimes the process may be slow and the underlying disorder go unrecognised for a long period. Heller's dementia in which psychosis develops during the fourth or fifth year of life belongs to this category. Chronic lead poisoning and brain damage as a result of encephalitis, may also produce psychotic pictures.

### Mental disturbance associated with psychosis in a caretaker

Rarely a child living in close contact with a psychotic adult, usually a parent, comes to accept the latter's delusions (false beliefs) and a situation comparable to *folie a deux* seen in adults develops. Generally this settles when the child is removed from the adult's care.

### Manic depressive psychosis

This is typically a disturbance of adult life characterised by periodic and profound changes of mood. It has seldom been reported in childhood (Anthony & Scott 1960), but the first episode may occur in adolescence, and is characterised either by severe depressive symptoms or by excitement and elation which are obviously abnormal.

### The autistic states

This largest group of serious mental disorders of childhood are of unknown aetiology, but have as a marked feature, a failure to relate to others in the environment. Because of this the word 'autism' has become strongly associated with them. Autism, which means to be withdrawn into oneself, may be used as an adjective, or as a noun as used by Kanner (1943) when he first described a subgroup of young psychotic children under the label of *early infantile autism*. Because autism is a characteristic of schizophrenia in adults, this has lead to the assumption that there is a relationship between these states and the schizophrenias of adult life. Studies by Kolvin and a group of workers in Britain (Kolvin *et al.* 1971) have clarified this relationship to some extent. A sample of eighty-three psychotic children were studied in detail. When they were ranked according to age of onset of the disturbance, it was found they fell into two definite clusters:

1   Those which began in the first three years of life and followed a chronic course. This disturbance was labelled *infantile psychosis* (I.P.) by Kolvin.

2   Those in which the disturbance began after the age of six years and followed a fluctuating course, called *late onset psychosis* (L.O.P.) by Kolvin.

In this series, only a very small number (3) became psychotic between the age of three and five years, and these all showed clearly recognisable degenerative disease of the central nervous system. Group 1 (I.P.) which had characteristics very similar to Kanner's Syndrome of infantile autism, showed no common features with schizophrenic illness in adults, and in one half at least there was strong suggestive evidence of neurophysiological dysfunction, possibly associated with cerebral damage in early life. Group 2 (L.O.P.) had some members which appeared to fall within the same biological continuum as adult schizophrenia. It is suggested that '*schizophrenia in childhood*' is reserved for these, and '*L.O.P. undifferentiated*' for the others. 'Childhood schizophrenia' is a confusing term and best not used.

The following Table 10.1, summarises our knowledge:

| Autistic states in childhood | | |
| --- | --- | --- |
| ONSET 0–3 YEARS | ONSET 5–6 YEARS | ONSET 7+ YEARS |
| *Early infantile autism* | Rare organic conditions, | *Late onset psychosis* |
| *Infantile psychosis*, strong | cerebral degenerations. | Some but not all resemble |
| suggestive evidence of | | schizophrenia in adults |
| neurological abnormality | | Reserve 'schizophrenia in |
| | | childhood' for those that |
| | | do. |

Let us now turn our attention to the clinical features of these two conditions. It is true that they are quite rare, but now the term 'autism' has entered common parlance, many parents seek their doctor's advice, fearing that some untoward behaviour in their child signifies the development of such a condition.

## EARLY INFANTILE AUTISM – INFANTILE PSYCHOSIS

### Onset

Behavioural abnormalities are recognised during the first three years of life. The mother complains her child is 'not cuddly', or is excessively irritable. Sometimes he is described as 'too good' in that he lies in his cot all day and makes no demands. Feeding difficulties are common.

### Symptomatology

It is generally accepted that three characteristics should be present in order to establish a firm diagnosis (Rutter 1974).

These are:

1 A failure to establish *social relationships*. The child isolates himself, avoids physical contact and eye-to-eye gaze. He prefers objects to people and may form abnormal attachments to these, often things which spin, such as fans or tops.

2 *Retardation of language development* with impaired comprehension. The child may remain mute or produce a few meaningless words. If speech develops, it is often used only to repeat what is said to him (echolalia), and not as a means of communication.

3 *Ritualistic and compulsive phenomena.* The child tries to preserve sameness in the environment, e.g. the same routine must be carried out every day. One child known to the author would only accept triangular sandwiches (any other shape upset him), and would spend hours observing them in different positions before he ate them. If play or routines are upset the child responds with anxiety and anger.

Other characteristics which are not exclusive to autism are:

● *Motor overactivity.* There is a lack of normal exploratory behaviour and this is replaced by aimless wandering and stereotyped, repetitive movements, e.g. finger flicking.

● *Sensory disturbances.* Some stimuli may produce a panic response, e.g. the child seems terrified of harmless objects, such as a vacuum cleaner, yet ignores painful stimuli or obvious danger.

● *Incomprehensible mood changes.* Rage or panic may occur without obvious cause. Self-mutilating behaviour can be very persistent, e.g. the child bites or scratches himself.

Originally autistic children were thought to be of good intelligence, but that this could not be accurately assessed because they related to others so poorly. Subsequently this was found not to be true. Many are mentally subnormal, however there is often wide variation among the skills of an individual. These children are not stigmatised in any way and look alert. This may belie their intellectual level. Sometimes exceptional skills, e.g. a phenomenal memory, are exhibited.

## Prevalence

Wing (Wing *et al.* 1967) studied a population of 8, 9 and 10-year-old children in the U.K. Two categories of autistic disorder were found:

1 *Nuclear autism,* which corresponded to the classical description by Kanner, and had an estimated prevalence of 2.1 in 10,000.

2 *Non-nuclear autism* in which some features of the condition were present. This had a prevalence rate of 2.4 in 10,000.

Thus, the overall prevalence of autistic conditions in childhood appears to be 4.5 in 10,000. Males outnumber females by 4 to 1. Kanner noted that a large proportion of the parents of autistic children came from social classes 1 and 2 (managerial or professional occupations). This phenomenon has been confirmed by Lotter (Wing 1976). In his series 60% of the fathers belonged to these social classes. Several suggestions have been put forward to explain this, such as: (i) Educated parents push for a diagnosis other than mental subnormality, (ii) because perinatal care is better the sequelae of cerebral insult at that time are more subtle (iii) that the children are of better intellectual potential and less likely to show global and severe intellectual handicap. None of these explanations are very convincing. Although mental subnormality is not a cause of autism many subnormal children show autistic behaviour.

## Aetiology

Initially parental aloofness and mechanistic methods of management were blamed for the child's lack of interest in interpersonal relationships. However, the concept of the 'refrigerating' or 'schizogenic' mother has not stood the test of time and may have done considerable harm in producing guilt-ridden parents. If a mother's management is to blame, how is it that the condition is often present very early in life, and that siblings of the autistic child are seldom affected similarly? Creak & Ini (1960) have shown that it is the reaction to a very frustrating child which often makes parents appear abnormal. The frustration to which they are subjected was described poignantly by the mother of autistic twin boys (her only children). When her husband returned from work in the evening, only the dog showed any pleasure.

Neurological abnormalities have frequently been implicated as a basis for infantile autism.

● Several studies have reported an increased incidence of *pre- and perinatal complications* in the birth histories of autistic children as compared to control groups (Kolvin 1971).

● About one half autistic children show *focal neurological defects* (Rutter 1968).

● *Abnormal electroencephalograms* have been reported in as many as 60–85% of autistic children (Creak & Pampiglione 1969) and long term follow-up shows an increasing incidence of epilepsy with age among autistic individuals (Rutter 1970).

● Diseases such as *phenylketonuria and congenital rubella* (Chess 1971) show a significant association with autism and these are known to affect brain function.

● Neurophysiological studies have shown *differences in vestibular function* between autistic children and normal controls (Ornitz 1970).

The suggestion of neurological dysfunction in a large proportion of autistic children leads some clinicians to consider the disorder with other manifestations of M.B.D. (see p. 165). However, no satisfactory explanation has been made in neurological terms and it may well be that autism represents the interaction of both physiological and psychosocial factors.

When the autistic child's profile of disabilities are compared with those of children suffering from receptive language disability (congenital dysphasia), similarities emerge. Patterns of subtest scores on standard intelligence tests are much alike (Bartak *et al.* 1975). However autistic children generally have more severe and wider ranging defects. Current opinion favour a basic cognitive deficit which involves skills relevant to the use and understanding of all language as a basis for infantile autism (Rutter 1977).

### Treatment

Many methods have been tried. Often results were disappointing; the following have proved most effective:

● *Educational therapy* by teachers working under psychiatric supervision has proved the most satisfactory. The rationale being that the psychotic child has irreversible personality defects and an effort must be made to develop as fully as possible, areas which are least damaged. Emphasis is placed on teaching the child ways of communicating and improving his social skills by offering a system of rewards.

● *Parents need practical advice* in how to manage a (sometimes) very difficult child and to be taught methods of helping him develop basic social skills. Placement in institutions has a detrimental effect and a day centre where parents can receive guidance from the staff who teach their children, is the ideal.

● *Supportive psychotherapy* may be necessary to help parents cope with their feelings of guilt and helplessness.

● *Drugs* can be helpful in controlling the difficult behaviour and extreme restlessness some autistic children show, but they do not affect the basic disorder. Response tends to be idiosyncratic and a trial of one or other tranquilliser may be necessary before suitable medication is found.

### The outcome of infantile psychosis

Follow-up studies are hard to interpret since it is not always clear how severely a child was affected and what a 'successful' outcome denotes. Bender's figures are generally accepted (Shaw & Lucas 1970). These are:

● One third come to function as *severely subnormal individuals* and are generally placed in institutions.

● One third become *family invalids* or settle in institutions for higher grade defectives.

● One third make *a reasonable adjustment* to their environment, they obtain employment but often remain schizoid, shut-in personalities who relate poorly to others and lack social perception.

Important prognostic indicators of a successful outcome are the presence of useful language by the age of 5, and a testable IQ of 70 or above (Eisenberg 1968). There is no evidence that these children become schizophrenic in adult life, though it has been suggested that some adults diagnosed as suffering from simple schizophrenia may have been autistic children but the condition went unrecognised in early life (Stone *et al.* 1968).

## LATE ONSET PSYCHOSIS

These children show a period of comparatively normal development before their disturbance begins. The clinical picture differs from the infantile psychosis group (Kolvin 1971) as follows:

● The families from which these children come are more commonly from average or *lower social classes* and are characterised by the presence of members with eccentric, often schizoid personalities.

● Although there is a tendency toward intellectual dullness in this group they *are not as clearly characterised by low IQ's* as are the infantile psychotics in whom a high percentage function below IQ 70.

● They may show evidence of *hallucinations*, e.g. hearing their thoughts spoken aloud, and of delusions or false beliefs.

## Diagnosis

This can be difficult; although the onset may be acute, it is frequently insidious and hard to recognise. Commonly a shy, eccentric 'odd' child or adolescent becomes progressively more and more disturbed but it is hard to know whether this is a transient disturbance common at this period of life, or the start of psychotic illness. Kolvin describes the following features as characteristic of L.O.P. They are listed in order of frequency.

● *Auditory hallucinations*, frequently repeated mannerisms or posturing, and a tendency to reply to questions with partial answers.

● *Disorders of thought*, with rather bizarre associations or thought blocking with sudden interruptions in the flow of speech and evidence of delusions. Abnormalities in mood, blunting of emotional responses or perplexity and grimacing or jerky movements.

● *Failure to mix with peers*, avoidance of adults, ambivalent attitudes and obsessional behaviour.

The older the child the more complex the symptomatology, and, in many cases the closer the resemblance to schizophrenic illness in adults. The age of onset, the verbal ability and the intelligence of the child will all affect the clinical picture. These conditions are rarer than infantile autism.

## Treatment

Supportive psychotherapy, helping the child cope with his perplexity in response to the disturbing nature of his symptoms is important. Attention must be paid to the parents' problems and their bewilderment at the odd behaviour of their child. Because of the rarity of these conditions it is often hard to give satisfactory answers as to prognosis, but advice about day to day management can be most helpful. The child should be kept within the educational system if at all possible and liaison with teachers is essential. Antipsychotic (neuroleptic) drugs (see Appendix A), are of value and should be given on a long term basis.

## Prognosis

This is more favourable if the onset is acute and the child previously well adjusted, as opposed to an insidious onset in a shy and withdrawn personality.

## CLINICAL EXAMPLES

*Early infantile autism*

George was nearly 3 when his mother brought him for help. She had made a great effort to understand her child, but latterly his difficult behaviour had become too much for her. It was quite impossible to leave him with baby sitters and she felt 'very depressed' about his future. She reported as follows:

'Ever since he was born I've felt there was something wrong with his personality. I've never been able to cuddle him or get him to look at me. He looks quite normal (physically), but I feel there's something between him and me. I've a little girl (twenty months younger), and I have a marvellous time with her – a real mother–daughter relationship but it's never been like that with George. I can't get him to come to me, he's so cut off. If he wants anything he screams or gets hold of my hand to try and make me get it, but he's never really spoken. He made a few baby sounds when he was one year old, but they faded away. I know he's not deaf because he hears trains and aeroplanes before I do and gets excited. Lately he's said "oh dear" and "cheerio", but just to himself and it doesn't mean anything. He likes to be alone; he's not interested in his sister. He's obsessed with toy cars. He spins the wheels for hours, lines them up again and again, or pulls them apart then puts them together. He loves spinning things, fans, the lids of pans, even the top of his boiled egg. He likes a strict routine and becomes upset if it is altered. With water restrictions, during a drought, he had to be bathed in the sink instead of the large bath to which he was accustomed. He just went mad with this and screamed all the time. Shopping with him is an ordeal; he won't go in lifts, he's terrified of them and he has to go to shops in the same order otherwise he lies in the road and screams. I'm sure his intelligence is good, he's clever with his hands and can work the washing machine. He mostly sits quietly alone playing with his cars. He used to sit and rock himself for hours, or flick his fingers in front of his eyes or bang his head on the wall. I've tried to get him playing with other children, but it's no good.'

George was the first child of a well adjusted couple who had been married for two years at the time of his birth. His mother suffered from anaemia throughout pregnancy, at the thirty-fourth week became toxaemic and labour was induced at thirty-eight weeks. It was 'prolonged and difficult' due to malpresentation, however George presented no physical abnormality at birth.

Feeding was difficult from the start, he would cry, kick, suck erratically and then vomit. His mother became convinced she 'couldn't get through to him' by the time he was aged six months. She visited several Child Welfare Clinics but was reassured because of his normal physical progress. Finally she read an article relating to autistic children in the popular press; she described how she responded to this, 'as I read it I felt, that's my George exactly'.

## *Late onset psychosis*

Peter was the only child of a middle aged couple and conceived after many years of marriage. He was delivered by Caesarian section after a long and difficult labour. Developmental milestones were passed at the appropriate ages although he was thought to be 'rather slow' with speech.

At the age of 6 he was described by his teacher as a quiet, shy, anxious boy who tended to play by himself, but overall his behaviour did not cause concern. Progress at school was poor and at 8 years he was moved to a small private institution which catered for the intellectually handicapped. He was well accepted initially but patience wore thin over the next two years because of his lack of social niceties and propensity to draw trains, toilets, and animals with their bones showing, on any object which came to hand. When this extended to the school gateposts his parents were advised to seek help. At the age of 10 years his mother described his symptoms as follows:

● He's quite absorbed in himself, he'll watch other children but withdraws into his thoughts and won't join in games. He often seems to be listening to something and mutters to himself.

● He hates his routine being disturbed. If I alter the arrangement of objects in his room he panics. We can't take him to the sea because the seagulls flying over terrify him.

● He's got such funny habits, he smells everything you give him, and spends a lot of time feeling the textures of things, he loves velvet. He's always biting his wrists and they are quite scarred now.

● He's no idea how to behave in public. He used a bad word in Church then threw the collection plate and money all over the floor. He's very difficult if people visit our home, says rude things, or runs away and hides from them.

On examination Peter was physically healthy and well developed. His mental state was observed at intervals over the next 3 years. Spontaneous use of speech was rare but he often repeated questions addressed to him (echolalia). He made some progress with school work and played the piano learning passages by ear. On entering the clinic he would look anxiously at all electrical fittings – he seemed to have some private fears relating to them. It was hard to establish rapport with him and most information was obtained by observing his paintings of which he produced a large number. A glimpse of the bizarre world in which he lived is shown in Fig. 4.10. Chapter 4 (parachutists sitting on toilets). He also drew many pictures of fish and chip shops, depicting horrible massacres. Human figures were cut up by a circular saw and the remains crated and sent to heaven, at the top of the page. Understandably, when in the street, he refused to go anywhere near a fish and chip shop and would walk round several blocks to avoid one.

In spite of the devoted efforts of his parents, Peter made little progress and by the age of 14 years the clinical picture remained unchanged.

## BIBLIOGRAPHY

### References

ANTHONY J. & SCOTT P. (1960). Manic depressive psychosis in Childhood. *J. Child Psychol. & Psychiat.* **1**, 58.
BARTAK L., RUTTER M. & COX A. (1975). A comparative study of infantile autism and specific developmental receptive language disorder. 1. The children. *Brit. J. Psychiat.* **126**, 127–145.
CHESS S. (1971). Autism in children with congenital rubella. *J. of Autism and Childhood Schizophrenia* **1**, 33–47.
CREAK E.M. & INI S. (1960). Families of psychotic children. *J. Child Psychol and Psychiat.* **1**, 156–175.
CREAK M. & PAMPIGLIONE (1969). Clinical and EEG studies on a group of 35 psychotic children. *Dev. Med. Child Neurol.* **11**, 218–227.
EISENBERG L. (1968). Psychotic disorders in childhood. *In* R. Cooke, ed, *The Biologic Basis of Paediatric Practice.* New York, McGraw Hill, Inc.
KANNER L. (1943). Autistic disturbances of affective contact. *Nervous Child* **2**, 217–250.
KOLVIN I. *et al.* (1971). Studies in childhood psychoses. *Brit. J. Psychiat.* 118, 381–419.
  (a) KOLVIN I. *Diagnostic criteria and classification.*
  (b) KOLVIN I., OUNSTED C., HUMPHREY M. & McNAY A. *The phenomenology of childhood psychoses.*
  (c) KOLVIN I., OUNSTED C., RICHARDSON I.M. & GARSIDE R.F. *Family and social background in childhood psychoses.*
  (d) KOLVIN I., GARSIDE R.F. & KIDD J.S.H. *Parental personality and attitude and childhood psychoses.*
  (e) KOLVIN I., OUNSTED C. & ROTH M. *Cerebral dysfunction and childhood psychoses.*
  (f) KOLVIN I., HUMPHREY M. & McNAY A. *Cognitive factors in childhood psychoses.*

188 Chapter 10

ORNITZ E. (1970). Vestibular dysfunction in schizophrenia and childhood autism. *Comp. Psychiat.* **11**, 159–173.
RUTTER M. (1968). Concepts of autism. A review of research. *J. Child Psychol. & Psychiat.* **9**, 1–25. (*Annual Progress* Vol **2**, 1969).
RUTTER M. (1970). Autistic children – infancy to adulthood. *Semin. Psychiat.* **2**, 435–450.
RUTTER M. (1974). The development of infantile autism. *Psychological Medicine* **4**, 147–163.
RUTTER M. (1977). Infantile autism and other childhood psychoses in *Child Psychiatry: Modern Approaches.* ed. M. Rutter & L. Hersov. Oxford, Blackwell Scientific Publications, Ch. 30, p. 732.
SHAW C.R. & LUCAS A.R. (1970). 2nd ed. *The Psychiatric Disorders of Childhood*, London, Butterworths. p. 123.
STONE A., HOPKINS R., MAHNKE M., SHAPIRO D.W. & SILVERGATE H.A. (1968). Simple schizophrenia, syndrome or shibboleth. *Amer. J. Psychiat.* **125**, 305–312.
WING L. (1976). Epidemiology and theories of aetiology Ch. 3 *in* Wing L. ed. hood: a survey in Middlesex. *Brit. Med. J.* **3**, 389–392.
WING L. (1976). Epidemiology and theories of aetiology Ch. 3 *in* Wing, L. ed. *Early Childhood Autism*, 2nd ed. Sydney, Pergamon Press p. 67.

## General Reading

KOLVIN I. (1972). Infantile autism or infantile psychoses. *Brit. Med. J.* **3**, 753–755.
KOLVIN I. (1972). Late onset psychosis. *Brit. Med. J.* **3**, 816–817.
ORNITZ E.M. & RITVO E.R. (1976). The syndrome of autism: a critical review. *Am. J. Psychiat.* **133**, 6, 609–21.

*See Appendix B.

# Chapter 11
# Mental Subnormality

'How often . . . . . . . . . had she sat beside him
night and day, watching for the dawn of a mind
that never came: how had she feared, and doubted
and yet hoped, long after conviction forced itself
upon her . . . . . . . . . . how, in the midst of all, she
had found some hope and comfort in his being
unlike another child, and had gone on almost
believing in the slow development of his mind
until he grew a man, and then his childhood was
complete – and lasting.'

Charles Dickens (1812–1870) Barnaby Rudge
(Jones 1972).

## GENERAL CONSIDERATIONS

It must not be forgotten that Child Psychiatric and Paediatric practice
involves work with the mentally subnormal. It includes the assessment of
skills and diagnosis of handicap, counselling families of retarded individuals and the management of behavioural and social problems if they
occur. The total management of the mentally subnormal child is best
handled by a team. Close liaison with psychologists, teachers and social
workers is essential.

### Definition

'Mental subnormality' is not a clearly defined entity but a heterogeneous
group of conditions characterised by low intelligence. 'Intelligence' is a
commonly used word but hard to define, and is usually described as the
*ability to adapt to new situations by means of purposeful thinking*. It refers
to the capacity to learn from experience and to apply such knowledge in
new and creative ways. Mental subnormality relates to conditions in
which there is retarded or arrested mental development present at birth
or in early childhood, and is thus distinct from dementia, in which a
deterioration of mental abilities occurs after a period of normal functioning.

## Classification of mental subnormality

This is based primarily on intellectual level (see Chapter 5), but factors other than intelligence should be considered when making a decision regarding the training of a subnormal individual. Within limits, stable personality traits and good social adjustment can be as important as intellectual level, in determining the child's eventual level of functioning.

The legal definition of mental subnormality applies to individuals with an IQ below 70, but the large group of individuals with an IQ between 70 and 85 are often labelled 'borderline' and may require special schooling.

The World Health Organization classifies degrees of mental subnormality as:

IQ  50–69  Mild subnormality
IQ  20–49  Moderate subnormality
IQ   0–19  Severe subnormality

The developmental characteristics which may be expected at these levels of intelligence are summarised in Table 11.1.

## Prevalence of mental subnormality

The inheritance of intelligence is thought to be polygenic and as with traits such as stature, its distribution follows a normal (Gaussian) curve. However, large populations show that the lower end of the curve departs from normality, and a disproportionate number of individuals fall below the level of IQ 45. It is thought that this is the result of the operation of single abnormal genes, and also 'reproductive casualties', i.e. abnormalities due to cerebral damage in the perinatal period.

## Is the prevalence of mental subnormality changing?

Studies such as that by Goodman and Tizard (1960) have shown that although there is an increased survival rate among the moderately and severely retarded (IQ below 50), the overall prevalence rate has declined.

TABLE 11.1.

## THE DEVELOPMENTAL CHARACTERISTICS OF THE MENTALLY SUBNORMAL

| Type of Subnormality | Pre-school Age 0–5 Yrs | School Age/Adolescence 6–20 Yrs | Adult 21+ Yrs |
|---|---|---|---|
| Mild | Able to develop social skills and to learn to communicate by speech. Motor development approximates normal. The handicap may not be recognised until a later age. | Needs to go at a slower pace than normal at school. May achieve grades 5 to 6 by teens. | Can achieve economic independence or attend a sheltered workshop. Requires support and guidance when faced with stress. |
| Moderate | Learns to communicate at a simple level. Requires supervision, and is able to profit from social training. Motor development may be fairly good. | Can be trained in social and occupational skills. Not likely to progress beyond grade 2 work at school at upper levels. Unable to cope with school work at lower levels. | Can perform unskilled or semi-skilled work under sheltered conditions only. Needs support and guidance when faced with mild stress. Can function well socially, but requires supervision. |
| Severe | Poor motor development. Unable to profit from training in self help. Very little communication possible. Lower grades need continual nursing care. | May develop limited communication skills. Benefits from habit training in upper grades, unable to do so in lower. | At upper level may learn some skills and is able to protect himself against environmental danger, but requires supervision and a controlled environment. Lower levels require constant nursing care. |

It seems that public health measures and advances in obstetrics and child care are responsible for this, in spite of the fact that they increase the chances of survival of the handicapped.

*Factors involved in prevalence studies*

It is generally estimated that 2–3% of the population are mentally subnormal, but these figures vary with the criteria used for selection and the facilities for detection of retardates. Five percent of all children born are potentially mentally subnormal (Slater & Roth 1969) but some suffer from conditions incompatible with life for more than a few weeks or months.

When broken down into age groups, the percentages of retarded in the population are found to be as follows:

   0– 6 years – 1%
  6–16 years – 3%
    16 years – 1%

The peak during childhood reflects the fact that many cases are not picked until school work is attempted. The apparent decline in incidence with age is because many retarded adults are self-supporting and socially well adjusted, and their handicap goes unnoticed.

Most (87%) mentally subnormal individuals fit into the range of mild retardation (IQ 50–69). They function well in the community and many are self-supporting, although they may need guidance at times of social or emotional stress. The majority of the remaining 13% can remain with their families, and commendable efforts are made nowadays to integrate them into the community. About 4% are severely retarded or show behavioural disturbance and require institutionalisation, as may those whose families are incapable of supporting them.

## AETIOLOGY

Most textbooks relating to intellectual handicap contain lists of possible aetiological factors and the student is referred to these for details. A summary of some likely causes follows. It should be remembered that it is quite possible for two or more factors to interact in one individual.

## Familial–cultural retardation

Most cases of mild mental retardation belong to his group and, as stated above, the mildly retarded comprise over three quarters of the total population of the intellectually handicapped. There is considerable evidence that a poor cultural environment retards intellectual growth. Programmes offering a stimulating environment to young children have resulted in substantial improvements in intellectual functions. Children of the poor are known to have a higher incidence of prematurity and difficult births. Malnutrition is frequent, as are infections which are often inadequately treated. Families are often unstable and emotional ties frequently disrupted. All these elements can contribute to intellectual deficiency, particularly if the individual has a relatively low innate intelligence which makes him less resistant to adverse circumstances, and the syndrome of familial–cultural retardation is probably the result of the interaction of several of these factors.

## Chemical agents

The ingestion of drugs e.g. thalidomide, during pregnancy, can produce physical handicap; to what extent they can produce intellectual deficiency is unknown. Heavy metals are known to produce mental handicap in young children who ingest lead through mouthing toys or other objects covered with paint containing lead.

## Physical factors

Ionising radiation is known to damage the foetal brain. This was shown following the Hiroshima bomb. The relationship between preconceptual irradiation of the gonads and mental retardation is still a matter for debate.

## Infections

Rubella, syphilis and toxoplasmosis in the prenatal period have all been implicated as precursors of mental deficiency. Bacterial meningitis and viral encephalitis may produce brain damage and intellectual handicap after birth.

*Prenatal and perinatal factors*

Relationships between the circumstances of birth and intellectual functioning are not entirely clear. However, low birth weight, maternal toxaemia, kernicterus following neonatal jaundice, and various conditions which reduce oxygen supply to the foetal brain are all suspect as regards mental handicap. Many parents of handicapped children give a history of adverse perinatal factors, but in some cases this may represent a need to resolve their own uncertainty rather than relate to fact.

*Nutrition*

Animal experiments have shown that severe malnutrition may produce changes in the developing central nervous system. It is thought that in underdeveloped countries extreme degrees of starvation may account for mental retardation.

*Inborn errors of metabolism*

Hereditary metabolic defects associated with a lack of specific enzymes due to the inheritance of rare autosomal recessive genes probably account for 3–5% of the retarded. Improved biochemical screening may uncover more. Phenylketonuria (P.K.U.) is a typical example, as is galactosaemia which consists of the inability to convert galactose to glucose.

*Degenerative diseases of the central nervous system*

Degenerative diseases of the central nervous system associated with the accumulation of lipoid substances in the cortex produce a gradual deterioration of intellect. These conditions are also associated with congenital enzymatic deficiency.

*Chromosomal abnormalities*

Mongolism (Down's syndrome) occurs approximately once in 700 births and is recognisable at birth. Maternal age is a major factor. After the age of 30 years the likelihood of mongol birth is multiplied 20 to 30 times, and the peak incidence in maternal age is reached between 45–49 years. The reason for this is not known, but the fundamental characteristic has been shown to be a chromosome abnormality. In over 90% this is due to the presence of a small extra chromosome making a complement of 47 instead of the normal 46 (trisomy 21, i.e. 3 of chromosome 21 instead of the normal 2). In the remaining 10% there is still an excess of genetic material, but the greater part of the extra chromosome is fused on to another chromosome producing an abnormally large one (translocation 15/21). Chromosomal abnormalities may occur in other groups, including the sex chromosomes, and be associated with mental subnormality.

### Endocrine deficiency

Cretinism, which is associated with defective thyroid function, is a rare cause of mental handicap.

### Pseudo-retardation

Children with primary physical defects, such as deafness or cerebral palsy, may be erroneously regarded as subnormal. If the basic condition is not diagnosed promptly and treated, they may eventually come to function at a retarded level.

## CONDITIONS ASSOCIATED WITH MENTAL SUBNORMALITY

### Autism

Not all autistic children are mentally subnormal, but many are, and it is not uncommon for the retarded child to show autistic behaviour (see p. 181).

### Epilepsy

Epilepsy is commoner among children suffering from intellectual handicap than in the normal population. Any damage to the brain may obviously produce both fits and limited intelligence. Idiopathic epilepsy, especially if it develops early in life, may produce brain damage itself, with the secondary development of mental subnormality.

## PSYCHIATRIC DISTURBANCE IN THE MENTALLY SUBNORMAL

It is generally recognised that the intellectually handicapped are more prone to develop psychiatric disturbance than normal individuals (Rutter *et al.* 1970). Possible reasons for this are:
- Organic brain disorder which may produce both intellectual handicap and behavioural disturbance.
- The child's response to stresses which inevitably accompany mental handicap.
- Adverse environmental factors such as parental instability, inconsistent management and poor physical care may prevent a child from making the best of his innate endowment as well as producing emotional disturbance.

Those who work with the handicapped have long recognised the need to supply additional support during periods of stress, for example when the individual first begins to live away from home or takes on a new job.

## ASSESSMENT OF THE MENTALLY HANDICAPPED

This should be along the following lines:
- *Medical history*. This should include enquiry as to possible aetiological factors, and a record of the age of passing developmental milestones.
- *Physical examination*. Neurological abnormalities and orthopaedic handicaps which may need correction should be noted. Vision and hearing must be checked. Audiometry is often necessary.
- A careful record should be made of current levels of *motor and language function and social development*.
- If *laboratory investigations* or E.E.G. are indicated, they should be instituted promptly.
- *Psychological assessment*. This should be performed by a psychologist experienced with the mentally handicapped. Often it is necessary, particularly in younger age groups, for the child to be seen for several sessions and over a period of time. Referral to education authorities for *advice about schooling* may be necessary.
- Investigation of the *social background*. This is generally done by a social worker and assessment made of the family's ability to cope with a handicapped member.

# HELPING THE PARENTS OF A RETARDED CHILD

To learn that their child is intellectually handicapped and unable to fulfil their expectations may be more grievous to parents than finding that he suffers from some chronic physical disease and may die. Supporting the parents of a retarded child requires skill, empathy and patience. When they first realise their child is developing slowly, many parents are emotionally unable to accept the implications. They often hope that the correction of a minor physical defect will provide a cure, or that he will grow out of it. Often they visit one agency after another in an attempt to gain a more favourable opinion.

When the diagnosis is given to parents, the emotional impact is such that they may be unable to comprehend what is said and it is essential that they be seen on several occasions and the nature of the condition gradually explained. They may find it hard to accept that in many cases the aetiology of mental handicap is unknown, and even the most unlikely suggestions they have as to aetiology, should be discussed seriously and sympathetically. The physician must not be offended if they ask for a second, or several opinions. Parents expect a thorough investigation of the child and any suggestions they have about this, providing they are not harmful, should be considered. Genetic counselling may be indicated, and in some cases referral to a specialist in this field may be necessary.

Sometimes parents have overoptimistic ideas about their child's level of intellectual functioning. In such cases 'sitting in' while the child is assessed by the psychologist can be most enlightening for them. It enables the psychologist to demonstrate to them what the child can and cannot do in comparison with others of his age.

Several studies have shown how inadequately the parents of handicapped children are managed. Hurtful and unnecessary words such as 'idiot' or 'moron' are sometimes used, or the diagnosis given abruptly and with minimal explanation. Parents must be given time to work through their feelings and to mourn the child that could have been. This process cannot be hurried. It is important for their adviser to guard against their developing an intolerant attitude, or feelings of guilt. The latter may cause them to focus all their attention on the retardate to the detriment of his siblings. Sometimes the handicapped child may be the result of an unwanted pregnancy and the mother may have quite irrational fears that her feelings of rejection toward him influenced his development. Occasionally she may have attempted to abort the pregnancy. Discussion of these private worries is of great value in coming to terms with the situation and in planning realistically for the future.

Parents of a handicapped child should be helped to realise that he has the same human needs as other children. Emphasis should be placed on his potential, what he can, rather than what he cannot do. Many parents ask whether the child should be placed in an institution. There is no doubt that in the early years there is no substitute for parental care. Providing the parents are given adequate support, and the family doctor is well placed to provide this, most parents cope very well. State services are able to organise short stay placements for the intellectually handicapped. This allows the handicapped child to become accustomed to going away, and gives the family an opportunity to pursue interests which they could not consider with the handicapped child at home. As time goes on, decisions have to be made as regards schooling. When puberty approaches, many parents worry about the possibility of uninhibited sexual behaviour. There is no evidence that sexual drive is increased in the mentally subnormal, but appropriate social behaviour may be learned only slowly. The provision of information and sympathetic guidance are perhaps even more important than with the normal child. Long term plans will include vocational training and perhaps placement in a hostel if the family are unable to supervise the retarded individual. Sometimes placement in an institution may be necessary as a permanent measure, depending upon the degree of handicap and the family's ability to cope with it.

# BIBLIOGRAPHY

## References

GOODMAN N. & TIZARD J. (1962). Prevalence of imbecility and idiocy among children. *Brit. Med. J.* **1,** 216–219.
JONES P.J. (1972). Dickens' Literary children. Harry Swift Memorial Lecture, *Aust. Paed. J.* **8,** 233–45.
SLATER E. & ROTH M. (1969). *Clinical Psychiatry.* 3rd ed. London, Balliere Tindall and Cassell. p. 694.
RUTTER M., TIZARD J. & WHITMORE K. (1970). *Education Health & Behaviour.* London, Langmore Group Ltd. Ch. 7.

## General Reading

CLARKE A.M. & CLARKE A.D.E. (1965). *Mental Deficiency, The Changing Outlook.* London, Methuen.
PENROSE L.S. (1972) *The Biology of Mental Defect.* 4th ed. London, Sidgwick and Jackson.

# Chapter 12
# Adolescence

'It's as large as life and twice as natural.'

Lewis Carroll (Charles Lutwidge Dodgson) 1832–1898
*Through the Looking Glass.*

This transitional stage between childhood and adult life has rather indefinite boundaries, but for practical purposes, adolescence can be regarded as the *second decade of life*; starting with onset of pubertal changes (acceleration in growth and the development of secondary sexual characteristics) and ending as the individual achieves sufficient maturity to deal with the realities of life by himself and to be responsible for himself and his actions. Individuals vary as to when physical changes start, but in general, girls are about two years ahead of boys.

Adolescence is popularly equated with emotional upheaval and rebellion, and sudden changes of mood, shifting ideologies and clashes with authority are universal. However, most youngsters and their parents make the necessary adjustments to allow a well balanced adult to emerge. If the child and his parents have coped with previous developmental stages successfully this augurs well for adolescence. If this is not the case, unresolved emotional difficulties from childhood may become reactivated or accentuated by the stress of adolescence.

## PSYCHOLOGICAL ASPECTS OF ADOLESCENCE

As in all phases of growth, the individual has certain 'tasks' to accomplish during adolescence. These are:

### Emancipation from parents

In order to achieve independence, the youngster must free himself from parental ties and learn to accept responsibility for himself. He will obtain support from his peer group as his dependency on parents wanes, and he must learn what responsibilities group membership entails. During the process of individuation he fluctuates between child-like dependency and stubborn independence and parents may find this most bewildering. Choice of a career involving tertiary education may mean financial dependence on parents long after emotional and physical maturity have been achieved. This does not always improve family relationships.

### Determination of sexual role

Heightened sexual impulses before personality structures are sufficient to contain them may result in episodes of uninhibited sexual behaviour. Homosexual activity may occur before the adolescent has sufficient confidence to approach members of the opposite sex, but this does not pressage a permanent homosexual orientation. Masturbation is almost universal among males and probably very common in females, although girls tend to be more secretive. 'Crushes' on older members of the same sex are very common and cannot be considered pathological.

Full adjustment to the sexual role is not always easy if there have been early identificatory difficulties, e.g. the tomboy girl who denies her femininity. Advanced or delayed pubertal changes in relation to contemporaries may be hard to accept. The boy whose sexual development is advanced or the girl who menstruates at 8 or 9 may be seriously embarrassed, as may those in whom pubertal changes are delayed. Even in these enlightened times some adolescents are ill prepared for puberty. The family doctor can be of great assistance to both the youngster and his parents, by offering reassurance if aspects of development are thought to be abnormal.

### Adjustments to body changes generally

Rapid physical growth may produce clumsiness – the youngster seems to have no control of his ungainly limbs. Discrepancies in the rate of growth at this age account not only for sports injuries among those who lag behind, but embarrassment on the part of those who come at either end of the continuum. Acne vulgaris may produce misery out of proportion to its extent. The sufferer may feel disfigured and withdraw from social relationships, or relate it to sexual acitivities or see it as punishment. Obesity is not uncommon, particularly among girls. Because this often relates to underlying personality difficulties (Bruch 1974), the girl must be helped with these, and dieting only started when she is emotionally able to accept it.

## Emotional development

The adolescent is typically ambivalent. He rebels against adult control, yet he wants guidance. He will test out authority figures to see how far he can go for he needs limits in order to feel secure. Sudden fluctuations in mood are common and may underlie much erratic behaviour. Internal controls are sometimes unable to cope with developing instinctual drives and uninhibited sexual behaviour (already described), episodes of aggression or gluttony may occur. The adolescent fears this loss of control and tries to defend himself by adopting attitudes of exaggerated aestheticism (retreat into purity), or intellectualism, becoming excessively involved in reading and thinking or debating, rather than actually seeking life experiences himself. Appearance, physiological functions, relationships with others and vocational choice may cause the individual much worry, and he is often too shy to discuss these with others. He hides his anxiety behind a facade of indifference, or hostility which cause him to be rejected and this impairs communication further.

## Intellectual development

The new-found ability to think logically causes the adolescent to indulge in incessant arguments and mental gymnastics of all kinds. Ruthless logic used to criticise the adult-made world he sees about him does not endear him to elders. As horizons widen, he comes to question family attitudes he accepted as a matter of course during childhood. He learns of his parents' human failings and is disillusioned to find they accept double standards of conduct.

## Social adjustment

The individual must find his identity as a person. The peer group plays an important part in socialisation, giving experience in the development of loyalty and social interaction. The adolescent's self concept is gradually acquired as the result of the reactions of his peers towards him. Initially, peer groups are the same sex, later they enlarge and include both sexes, offering opportunities for heterosexual experience. Conformity to the

group in both appearance and behaviour becomes tremendously important. Sometimes gangs indulge in types of antisocial behaviour, which
they would not consider as individuals. Lack of money to indulge in a
popular 'craze' may cause unhappiness and sometimes thieving. The
working adolescent has a relatively large pay packet and is often exploited
by commercial interests to the extent that he is unable to cope with the
situation.

Choice of a vocation may be forced upon an individual before he is
ready. Some youngsters enter educational courses or apprenticeships
which are inappropriate and experience failure, sometimes a series of
failures. School counsellors and vocational guidance bureaux have an
important part to play in helping them avoid these mistakes.

In summary, adolescence is a period of rapid *physical* and *psychological*
growth, during which the individual must establish his *identity* and find
his *social, sexual* and *vocational roles* in the society to which he belongs.
At a time of rapid social change and when considerable demands are
made upon youth, it is not surprising that some show signs of emotional
difficulties. It is probably a reflection on the resilience of human personality that many weather the storm so well.


## PARENTS OF ADOLESCENTS

Parental fears for the child in today's permissive society are often realistic,
yet attempts to restrict activities are met by resentment because the
adolescent feels he is not being allowed the same degree of freedom as his
peers. Some parents condone uninhibited behaviour in childhood,
laughing it off as a sign of high spirits, but become seriously concerned
when it is carried over into adolescence and shown by an individual with
an adult's physical strength and drives. They slowly become aware that
their mistakes have come home to roost. Parents who have been frustrated
in their own careers may have unrealistic expectations for their children.
This may come to a head when a career choice has to be made, and the
youngster may be forced into a vocational training in which he is unlikely
to succeed. Adolescent behaviour may reactivate conflicts relating to a
parent's own adolescence; thus a parent whose adolescence was unduly
restrictive may unconsciously encourage his child's antisocial behaviour,
and derive vicarious pleasure from the escapades.

Psychiatric disturbance in parents will have considerable impact on
the emotional development of the adolescent. For example, a neurotic

mother may be incapable of giving her child freedom to grow up; a depressed parent will find it hard to cope with adolescent exuberance.

## PREVALENCE OF PSYCHIATRIC DISTURBANCE IN ADOLESCENCE

Epidemiological studies of disturbance in adolescence in Australia show that about 15% have significant psychiatric symptoms (Stoller 1972). Since adolescents constitute 15% of the Australian population, this means that nearly one quarter of a million in this age group require some degree of psychiatric help. Treatment facilities for adolescents are generally not well developed in this country, and there is a great need for the establishment of inpatient and outpatient units able to deal with their specific problems.

## TYPES OF PSYCHIATRIC DISTURBANCE IN ADOLESCENCE

### *Adaption (situational) reactions*

Stresses to which the adolescent in Western society is subjected are described above, and relate to:
● Developmental change, physical and psychological.
● The need to find a role in society.
● Family disturbance.
   Individual vulnerability to stress varies considerably but a carry over of childhood difficulties impairs the adolescent's ability to cope with stress at a level appropriate to his age.
   The symptomatology of stress reactions is, very wide. Common manifestations which parents (and others) complain about are:
● Aggressive, antisocial acting-out behaviour.
● Anxiety, moodiness, and social withdrawal.
● Failure at school or work which is often seen as 'laziness'.
   Occasionally the disturbance may be such to raise the question of serious mental illness. Hopefully most episodes are benign and settle as pressures ease or the individual matures sufficiently to be able to withstand stressful situations. Episodes of acutely disturbed behaviour are sometimes labelled 'adolescent turmoil' – this is not, a nosological entity.

## Neurosis

Neurotic symptoms may develop de novo or be carried over from childhood.
● *Anxiety* may be hidden behind a facade of indifference or aggression. Acute anxiety amounting to a state of disordered panic may appear in a background of chronic anxiety, and is often related to sexual problems, particularly to homosexuality.
● *Phobias.* These may relate to disease, germs, travelling alone or mixing with crowds. School phobia at high school age is of more serious import than in the early years (see p. 109).
● *Obsessional behaviour.* The individual may have shown obsessional traits in childhood or his symptoms appear for the first time at puberty. If severe, compulsive rituals may incapacitate the sufferer at school or at work.
● *Conversion reactions* are perhaps not as common as they were a few generations ago, however paralyses, disturbances in vision, or fainting attacks' may occur.
● The question of *depression* occurring as a clinical entity in young people has already been raised in Chapter 7. In the younger adolescent depression is often expressed indirectly, with complaints of boredom or restlessness. The patient sees himself as inferior, or the world as being all wrong. Somatic symptoms, pains, aches and headache are common. Sometimes antisocial behaviour may be a presenting feature. In the older adolescent, depressive illness comes to resemble that in adults, especially when the individual develops the insight and verbal ability necessary to describe his feelings of hopelessness and guilt. Usually adolescent depression is part of a neurotic disturbance, but in the later years of adolescence, depression may reach psychotic dimensions, and sometimes a depressive episode may herald the onset of manic-depressive illness.

## Personality disorder

As in childhood, personality disorders are not often diagnosed in early adolescence. However, in the later years, abnormal traits may become sufficiently prominent to warrant their acceptance as a permanent feature. Persistent delinquent acts always raise the question of a developing sociopathic personality (see p. 114) but we are not at the stage of being able to recognise with certainty features likely to pressage the development of adult psychopathy. Homosexual behaviour is not uncommon especially in institutional settings where heterosexual outlets are limited, but generally, this is outgrown.

## Anorexia nervosa

This is seen typically in adolescent girls, the usual age of onset being 14-18 years, and has a prevalence rate of up to 1% in girls of 16 years and over. A similar condition is recognised much less frequently in males. It appears to be increasing in Western Society (Crisp *et al.* 1976). It is characterised by:

● A persistent refusal to eat. The girl is not anorexic and may indulge in bouts of overeating followed by self-induced vomiting; she is determined to remain thin and will eat and retain only as much as is consistent with that aim.

● A coexistent endocrine disturbance manifested primarily by amenorrhoea.

● A history of mild obesity and the start of a weight reducing programme which progresses to an aversion to food in a family which is often food oriented.

### Physical features

● The patient is excessively thin with reduced basal metabolic rate, bradycardia, acrocyanosis, and a growth of downy hair over the skin (lanugo) may develop.

● Energy is unimpaired and the girl continues with her normal activities quite unconcerned about her physical state. Often she busies herself preparing food for others.

### Psychopathology

● The condition appears to arise out of a conflict situation associated with growing up and assuming the mature sexual role.

● Emotional immaturity is marked and the girl generally has an ambivalent relationship with her mother who is made acutely anxious by the loss of weight. Obsessional traits are common.

● The syndrome may be seen as a neurotic disorder with a phobic reaction to the changes of puberty and a distorted perception of an ideal weight for age, leading to a refusal to eat and grow larger, with secondary hypothalamic dysfunction.

*Differential diagnosis*
● Psychiatric illness, such as depression with secondary anorexia.
● Physical illness, such as malabsorption syndrome, tuberculosis, malignancy or hypopituitarism.

*Management*
● These patients cannot be trusted and will adopt any subterfuge to avoid a gain in weight.
● All but the mildest cases should be admitted to hospital under close supervision.
● The attendant must not be manipulated into filling the mother's role of continually coaxing the patient to eat. It must be explained to the patient that she is responsible for gaining weight, and a contract made that when a given target is achieved she will be allowed certain privileges. Bed rest should be instituted at the start with progressive removal of restrictions dependent upon weight gain.
● A liquid diet providing 2,000 calories a day may gradually be replaced by high calorie solid food, the aim being for an intake of 3,000–5,000 calories per day.
● Psychotherapy with the patient, exploring and attempting to resolve her unhealthy attitudes toward growing up is important. Work with her family is essential.
● Tube feeding is only necessary if the patient's condition causes serious concern.
● Phenothiazines may be of help in overcoming the resistance to eating, e.g. chlorpromazine up to 600 mg/day may be given.

*Prognosis*
● The patient is likely to require psychiatric supervision for a long period. Relapses are not uncommon. Death, from suicide or inanition may occur.
● Long-term studies have shown that about half the patients remain underweight and social and sexual difficulties commonly persist. A smaller proportion may continue to show menstrual irregularities.

*Psychosis*

*Schizophrenia.* Emotional upheavals are common during adolescence but if a seriously disturbed adolescent does present, the possibility of psychotic illness must always be kept in mind. Schizophrenia is a serious mental illness which occurs with increasing frequency during adolescence and early adult life. The aetiology is unknown; as a working hypothesis it can be considered to result from a genetic predisposition *plus* environmental stress, which may be physical or psychological. It may well represent a group of illnesses with symptoms in common. These are as follows:

● The youngster gives vague answers with attention to unimportant detail Conversation fails to progress in logical sequence (*thought disorder*). At the end of the interview, one is left with the feeling that it has led nowhere.

● There is *blunting of emotional responsiveness* and although the patient generally appears callous and unfeeling, there may be sudden episodes of rage or fear. Emotional display is often inappropriate to the accompanying thoughts (*incongruity of affect*). It is difficult to establish rapport with the patient.

● The adolescent becomes apathetic, withdrawn and involved in his own thoughts, *i.e. autistic*. He may show persistent negativism.

● *Delusions and hallucinations* are common. A delusion is a false belief which is maintained fixedly in the face of reason. A hallucination is a sensory perception which occurs in the absence of external sensory stimulation. Hallucinations may occur in any sensory modality, but are commonly auditory.

The two clinical varieties of schizophrenia commonly seen in adolescence are:

(i) Hebephrenic type, in which the patient shows rather florid symptoms as described above. Typically he presents a silly, giggling manner, unpredictable, inappropriate behaviour and grossly disordered thinking.

(ii) Simple type, which is characterised by an insidious withdrawal from interpersonal relationships, failure at school or work, apathy and aimlessness. More florid positive symptoms develop much later.

The other varieties of schizophrenia, i.e. catatonic and paranoid, are rare in early adolescence.

The onset of schizophrenia may be acute or slowly progressive. An acute onset in an adolescent who has a good premorbid personality, and when there is some definite precipitating cause, has a reasonably good prognosis. Complete recovery may occur, or recovery with minimal personality deterioration. A gradual onset in an individual with a long history of social isolation and eccentricity carries a poor prognosis, and the patient likely to become a chronic psychiatric invalid who requires institutionalisation.

*Manic depressive psychosis*. This is also a severe mental illness, characterised by alternating periods of depression and mania (a state of euphoria hyperactivity and excitement); it is much less common in this age group than is schizophrenia. However, the first manic or depressive episode may be recognised in the older adolescent.

*Psychosis associated with known brain pathology.* Transient psychoses may develop in association with drug abuse or encephalitis or following head injury, but for practical purposes, in the acutely psychotic adolescent the diagnosis rests between schizophrenia and drug induced psychosis.

### Chronic brain syndromes

Head injuries due to traffic accidents are an increasing problem in this age group; sequelae include intellectual deficit, loss of previously acquired skills, and (often a major difficulty) the development of disinhibited behaviour.

*Management includes:*
- Adequate assessment of intellectual, physical and behavioural status prior to discharge from hospital.
- Rehabilitation and vocational training.
- Control of disinhibited behaviour in so far as this is possible by giving advice and support to the family or caretakers, and use of medication.
- Attention to neurological sequelae such as epilepsy.

## PHYSICAL HANDICAP IN ADOLESCENCE

As noted in Chapter 8, children generally adapt well to physical handicaps especially if these are present from birth or develop early in life. With the approach of adolescence and a growing realisation of what a given handicap entails, attitudes may change. Interference with peer group activities, sporting committments and above all interaction with the opposite sex may occasion much anger and resentment. Sometimes the adolescent may refuse to carry out treatment ordered for a physical condition as a means of expressing his rebellion. Sometimes, he blames his parents for his handicap and expresses the resentment he feels toward them. Many youngsters with handicaps see the future stretching interminably ahead with no prospect of compensation for their suffering. Group therapy will often help these patients especially if interaction with others of the same age with physical handicaps can be arranged. Teaching the youngster to capitalise on his potential and develop skills in areas not affected by his handicap is important. Enrolment with an association organised for the sufferers of a specific handicap can also be helpful.

# DRUG ABUSE IN ADOLESCENCE

There is no need to stress the importance of this problem today. Figures relating to prevalence are understandably hard to obtain but there can be few youngsters who have not had contact with others using drugs or have not experimented themselves. The adolescent culture lends itself to group activities and these include 'mind expanding' experiences such as drug taking, or investigation into the occult.

## Factors predisposing to drug abuse

There is no specific personality type. Any youngster who feels a misfit has difficulty with interpersonal relationships, lacks the support of his family and looks for acceptance into a group which indulges in drug abuse is at risk. So too, is the individual who looks for a means of gaining confidence or because he is bored or craves excitement. Drugs may be taken as a gesture of rebellion. The example set by many adults who are dependent upon alcohol or barbiturates does not help the situation.

## Types of drugs

The drugs used are constantly changing. Some youngsters will try anything likely to produce psychic effects. The large numbers of pills available in homes today make experimentation all too easy. Antihistamines have had a recent vogue. Common drugs used may be classified according to their effects:
1    C.N.S. depressants
    Alcohol
    Barbiturates and other hypnotics and sedatives
    Narcotic analgesics – heroin
        morphia
        opium
        methadone
        pethidine
2    C.N.S. stimulants
    amphetamines
    methylphenidate
    cocaine

3  Hallucinogens
   L.S.D. (lysergic acid diethylamide)
   psilocybin
4  Cannabis
   which has properties common to all the above and is the most widely
   used.

Individual reactions to a drug vary depending upon the dose, the affective state prior to taking the drug, and the social setting in which it is taken.

Drugs are obtained from friends, by theft, misrepresentation to doctors and forged prescriptions. The need for money to buy drugs may underlie some juvenile crime and prostitution. Cannabis grows only too easily in Australia and fungi containing psilocybin occur naturally. L.S.D is often home made and of variable strength and may contain impurities.

A popular method of producing 'kicks' is by inhalation of gaseous substances. Dry cleaning fluid (carbon tetrachloride), petrol, volatile adhesives (model airplane cement) and various aerosols (e.g. hair spray) are frequently used. Death can result from the direct effects of an extremely toxic substance or through suffocation because the substance is inhaled using a plastic bag and the individual loses consciousness.

## Patterns of drug use

Whether the use of cannabis leads to the taking of other drugs is debatable. Social and environmental factors are of greater importance than any inherent properties of a drug. However, a common sequence of events is from cannabis to the hallucinogens which may then be supplemented by narcotics or more rarely cocaine.

## Detection

Parents often ask a doctor by what means they may recognise their child is taking drugs. Moodiness, social withdrawal, a neglected appearance and deterioration in school work are not uncommon events in adolescence and do not necessarily indicate drug abuse.

● A careful clinical history is of the greatest value. The youngster enjoys his activities and is likely to be resentful if anyone attempts to deprive him of his pleasure. It will require time and patience to establish worthwhile communication with him, and only when this has been done will any admission as to the use of drugs be forthcoming.

- There may be a history of episodes of overexcitability or drowsiness.
- The only really useful physical signs are sores and needle marks over the course of veins.
- Urine analysis can detect most drugs used today, but this requires specialised laboratory facilities.

## Management

*Acute.* A 'bad trip' occurs when a hallucinogen alters perception and feeling to the extent that the individual becomes acutely disturbed. Removal of excited companions and calm reassurance that the effects will pass of, i.e. 'talking the patient down', is the correct approach. Because external stimuli are magnified and distorted, a quiet atmosphere is essential. Medication is generally not recommended, unless the disturbance is severe when diazepam (intravenously or by mouth) should be used. Cannabis intoxication should not require medication.

*Long-term.* Once initial contact is made, it is essential to assess how much involvement with drugs has occurred and what psycho-social factors operate. Frank discussion of the dangers of drug abuse; arranging environmental change when necessary, support and careful follow-up, may be possible in a general practice setting, but frequently referral to a clinic specialising in these problems is necessary.

## Prevention

- Adolescents seldom need psychoactive drugs. If medication is necessary e.g. in anxiety states or sleep disturbance, drugs should be prescribed for short periods only.
- If drugs are prescribed for older members of the family, they should be warned of the dangers of leaving them around the house.
- Doctors should be on the alert for thefts of pills and prescription pads.
- Some youngsters are remarkably clever in producing 'symptoms'. Doctors should beware of being tricked into prescribing for these.

## SUICIDE IN ADOLESCENCE

In the past there has been a lack of recognition of the extent to which suicidal behaviour occurs in late childhood and early adolescence (*Brit.*

*Med. J.* 1975). Suicide ranks fourth as the leading cause of death in the fifteen to nineteen age group (Toolan 1974), surpassing deaths from tuberculosis, leukaemia and all contagious diseases. It has been estimated that nearly fifty percent of suicides are disguised as accidents; this is especially the case in young people whose families react with shame (and sometimes guilt about their contribution to the problem), and attempt to deny the reality of the situation. Males outnumber females *in deaths by suicide* at all ages and in all cultures. *Suicide attempts*, however, show a very marked reverse in sex ratio to this. Toolan (1974) reports it to be of the order of seven females to one male. Thus during adolescence a continuum of suicidal behaviour exists: on one hand the histrionic girl who reacts to minimal frustration with a minor self injury, on the other a boy who makes a determined effort to kill himself. Although depression may be the basis for suicide, there are often other motives, such as a desire for revenge ('You'll be sorry for treating me badly when I'm dead'), a 'cry for help', or the wish to join a dead relative. Occasionally suicidal behaviour may herald a schizophrenic breakdown.

Many adolescents seem not to recognise the full implications of suicide. Even if they do, they are so overwhelmed by their emotions they make a serious attempt on the spur of the moment. Suicidal behaviour in young people must be taken seriously. Admission to hospital protects the patient against further efforts to harm himself and allows assessment of him and his parents. There is usually an underlying family problem and work with the child within the context of his background is essential.

## SCHOOLGIRL PREGNANCIES

Pregnancy in the early teens is on the increase and becoming a worldwide problem (*Brit. Med. J.* 1975). It often appears within the context of feelings of rejection and rebellion in the girl, and represents for her a disruption in schooling, interference with her choice of vocation and exposure to the psychological effects of termination or a decision about the future of her child before she is mature enough to make it. For the baby there is the increased likelihood of perinatal complications (*Brit. Med. J.* 1976), neglect, and sometimes cruelty (child abuse). Therapeutic abortion in early adolescence can be followed by feelings of guilt, anger and depression (Perez-Reyes & Falk 1973), but these appear in the immediate post-operative period and their duration and intensity relate indirectly to the support given to the mother. Most girls experience the 'crisis' and operation as part of the process of growing up and return to function well in school and in society if offered help, rather than criticism and punishment. Should the pregnancy continue it is undoubtedly in the best interests of the child that it be adopted. Nevertheless the girl herself must be given an opportunity to decide whether or not she keeps her child and at this stage skilled counselling by a social worker is essential. A mother may suffer significant depression if she has not been given the opportunity to work through her feelings in relation to relinquishing her child to adoptive parents. There is much to be said for pregnant teenagers being managed as a separate group in obstetric clinics and hospitals; not only do they gain support from each other but they are protected from the criticism of older women. A major part of case management involves supervision of the girl's return to school and vocational training. There is evidence that delay in this respect may increase the risk of another conception.

Attention to *preventive measures* is most important. Health education in schools should include practical details of contraceptive methods and means of obtaining contraceptive advice – information which is often not forthcoming in the girl's family setting. Instruction must be geared to the needs of less intelligent girls who present a greater risk of pregnancy. This practical advice must of course, be given within the context of general sex education and of interpersonal relationships generally. The need of a counsellor in every secondary school to whom a girl can go for advice if she thinks she is pregnant, would seem obvious.

## MANAGEMENT OF THE DISTURBED ADOLESCENT

### *Interviewing adolescents*

Many people find communication difficult especially as the adolescent tends to identify authority figures with his parents (or others with whom he has clashed), and transfer his negative attitudes to the examiner. It is important not to allow any suggestion of 'taking sides' and often best to see the youngster first, so that he can state his case before his parents tell their story; or the family may be seen together.

Points to remember when talking to adolescents:

● *Absolute honesty is essential.* The patient should be told what is going on, as would be done with any responsible person. There must be no suggestion that he is being treated like a child.

● The examiner must *be his age* and not attempt to talk or behave as an adolescent. This approach will immediately be seen as phoney.

● The examiner must remember that the youngsters behaviour may *reactivate conflicts* relating to his own adolescence, making him unduly critical of, or ready to condone, certain aspects of his patient's behaviour.
● The adolescent's *ambivalent attitudes* and sudden changes of mood must be accepted. The examiner will find himself on a pinnacle at one time, despised at the next, but his should not alter the overall relationship, if it is handled with insight.
● Anyone working with adolescents must be prepared to *act as a good parent*. One who is sympathetic and consistent, but able to be firm. He must be prepared for the adolescent to 'test him out', in order to discover the limits of his tolerance, remembering that the youngster needs external controls in order to feel secure.

### Psychiatric emergencies in adolescence

Severe depression, acute anxiety states, adverse drug reactions (bad trips) and acute psychotic episodes may all require emergency treatment. Unless the cause is immediately obvious and remediable, e.g. a drug reaction which appears likely to settle, admission to hospital should be arranged in order to reach a firm diagnosis and to assess the background from which the individual comes.

Acute situational crises involving angry and aggressive behaviour on the adolescent's part may cause considerable disturbance in the casualty department. The cardinal principle is to find out what is going on and why the patient is so angry. A calm enquiry such as 'Why are you feeling like this ?' will often elicit a sensible reply, whereas admonitions to control himself and threats of physical restraint will often produce more aggression. The most churlish adolescent will usually respond to a sincere attempt to understand his view-point and time must be taken to help him realise his welfare is a primary consideration. Once rapport has been established, and the patient has been given time to cool down, plans should be made for long-term treatment and follow-up.

### Psychotherapy

Although individual psychotherapy has an important part to play, group therapy is particularly valuable at this age, utilizing the individual's natural motivation to rely on group support.

## Drug treatment

Drugs should always be used sparingly. Many adolescents will want 'to go it alone' and, indeed, it is generally far better that they should. The possibility of the development of drug dependence and of suicide must always be considered before prescribing.

## Social support

Hostel accommodation, vocational guidance, introduction to youth clubs and other group activities can be most important especially if the adolescent is shy or lacks social experience.

## The parents

As with younger children, the adolescent must be viewed within the context of the family setting. Assessment of parental disturbance may be a part of treatment. Psychiatric help for parents may have to be arranged.

# BIBLIOGRAPHY

## References

BRITISH MEDICAL JOURNAL (1975). *Editorial annotation.* Suicide in children **1**, 592.
BRITISH MEDICAL JOURNAL (1975). *Editorial annotation.* Pregnancy in Adolescence **3**, 665.
BRITISH MEDICAL JOURNAL (1976). *Editorial annotation.* School pregnancies **2**, 545.
BRUCH H. (1974). Eating disturbances in adolescence. In *American Handbook of Psychiatry.* 2nd ed. Editor S. Arieti. New York. Basic Books Vol **II** Chap. 18.
CRISP A.H., PALMER R.L. & KALUCY R.S. (1976). How common is anorexia nervosa. A Prevalence Study. *Brit. J. Psychiat* **128**, 549–54.
PEREZ-REYES M.G. & FALK R. (1973). Follow-up after therapeutic abortion in early adolescence. *Arch. Gen. Psychiat.* **28**, 120–126. (*Annual Progress* Vol **6**, 1974).
STOLLER A. (1972). Social Psychiatry and public health. *Aust. N.Z. J. Psychiat.* **6**, 1, 9–18.
TOOLAN J.M. (1974). Depression and suicide in adolescence. In *American Handbook of Psychiatry.* 2nd. ed. Editor S. Arieti. New York: *Basic Books Inc.* Vol **II**, Chapter 20.

## General reading

BEWLEY T. (1975). The illicit drug scene. *Brit. Med. J.* **2**, 318–320.

BOYD P. (1972). Emotional problems in childhood and adolescence. Adolescents –
   drug abuse and addiction. *Brit. Med. J.* **4**, 540–43.
BRITISH MEDICAL JOURNAL. (1971). *Editorial annotation.* Anorexia nervosa. **4**, 183.
BRITISH MEDICAL JOURNAL. (1972). *Editorial annotation.* Anorexia nervosa in
   males. **4**, 686.
GROUP FOR THE ADVANCEMENT OF PSYCHIATRY. (1968). *Normal Adolescence, Its
   Dynamics and Impact.* New York, Scribners.
HENDERSON A.S. (1969). The nature of adolescent psychiatric illness. *Aust. N.Z. J.
   Psychiat.* **3**, 120–123.
HOWELLS J.G. ed. (1971). *Modern Perspectives in Adolescent Psychiatry.* Edinburgh,
   Oliver & Boyd.
MEDICAL JOURNAL OF AUSTRALIA. (1973). *Editorial annotation.* The psychiatry of
   adolescence. **1**, 13, 621–622.
MEDICAL JOURNAL OF AUSTRALIA SUPPLEMENT (1974). *Problems of adolescence.* **1**, 4,
   19–26.

*See Appendix B.

# Appendices

## A. THE USE OF PSYCHOACTIVE DRUGS IN CHILDHOOD

### General principles

● Generally, drugs should be used as an adjunct to other methods of treatment such as psychotherapy or environmental manipulation (see p. 13).

● Their most effective use is for a short period (to break a vicious circle) e.g. to reduce restlessness or improve mood while other measures take effect.

● One drug at a time given an adequate trial as regards dose and period of administration is the correct approach. Apart from the management of epilepsy, polypharmacy is not indicated in childhood.

● It is better to use a small number of well known and well tried drugs regularly than to experiment with every new preparation that comes on the market.

● Children are suggestible, and their placebo response is high. Objective assessment of the effects of medication is essential, thus the report of a teacher can be very helpful. Parents emotional involvement with the child's difficulties may impair their judgement.

● It is well to make sure that parents *give* the child his tablets *and* that he swallows them.

● The reason for prescribing drugs should be explained to older children.

● Prescription of these drugs should be accompanied by a warning to keep them under lock and key.

### Drugs prescribed for children

These are listed below. The tables give the dose over 24 hours for a 10-year-old. A 5-year-old might be expected to take about one half of these doses. After 12 years, doses approximate those used for adults.

## NEUROLEPTICS: ANTIPSYCHOTICS: MAJOR TRANQUILLISERS I

These are used for severe behaviour disorders characterised by hyperactivity and aggression. They must never be used indiscriminately for behaviour problems; careful assessment of aetiological factors is essential in the first instance. There are few contraindications, side effects which include dystonic reactions and in the case of chlorpromazine, photosensitivity, are rarely a problem. Parenteral administration is very

TABLE A.1

## NEUROLEPTICS: ANTIPSYCHOTICS: MAJOR TRANQUILLISERS

| Name | Trade Name | Max. dose/24 hr for 10 year old |
|---|---|---|
| chlorpromazine | Largactil | 100 mg |
| thioridazine | Melleril | 100 mg |
| pericyazine | Neulactil | 25 mg |
| *trifluoperazine | Stelazine | 4–6 mg |
| *haloperidol | Serenace | 3–5 mg |

*May require concurrent administration of an anti-parkinsonian agent, e.g. benztropine mesylate (Cogentin) 2 mg/day if dystonic symptoms develop.

seldom indicated and should be reserved for hospital practice. The use of retard preparations is not advisable. Syrup preparations are used extensively because they are more palatable. However, some of the dose may be left on the spoon or container.

TABLE A.2

## MINOR TRANQUILLISERS

| Name | Trade Name | Max. dose/24 hr for 10 year old |
|---|---|---|
| diazepam | Valium | 10 mg |
| chlordiazepoxide | Librium | 10 mg |

These can be of value as a short term measure while other methods of treatment take effect, e.g. returning a phobic child to school, but there is much to be said for a child working through his anxiety in relation to a situation with the support of a therapist, rather than with the support of drugs. Diazepam is most generally used. Toxic effects are rare.

## ANTIDEPRESSANTS

Depressive illness is being recognized with increasing frequency in childhood. Supportive help and modification of the environment are of greater importance than drug treatment but, depending upon the severity of the symptoms, tricyclic antidepressants may be used. Where depression and anxiety coexist, amitriptyline which has both anxiolytic and antidepressant properties may be useful. For the treatment of bedwetting with tricyclic antidepressants (see p. 158).

TABLE A.3

## ANTIDEPRESSANTS (TRICYCLIC GROUP)

| Name | Trade Name | Max. dose/24 hr for 10 year old |
|---|---|---|
| imipramine | Tofranil | 100 mg |
| amitriptyline | Laroxyl, Tryptanol Saroten, | 100 mg |
| nortriptyline | Aventyl, Allegron Nortab | 100 mg |

Atropine-like effects may be noticed for a short period when these drugs are started, e.g. blurred vision or drowsiness. Members of this group are very dangerous if an overdose is taken.

Antidepressants of the manoamine oxidase inhibitor group are very seldom used in childhood; for details of their administration the reader should consult texts relating to the Psychiatry of Adults.

## HYPNOTICS AND SEDATIVES

Psychiatric disturbance in childhood may be associated with a disturbed sleep pattern; generally this settles when treatment is directed toward the basic problem. If hypnotics are required nitrazepam (Mogadon) 2.5–5 mg. a night or triclofos (given as Tricloryl Syrup up to 10 ml a night) are both useful. In infancy and early childhood disorders of sleep require a review of daytime management and parent attitudes, rather than medication. If a hypnotic is used, it should only be given for a short period to re-establish a regular pattern. Promethazine (Phenergan) 5–10 mg given in an elixir containing 5 mg/5 ml may be used.

Apart from the treatment of epilepsy barbiturates should be avoided with younger children who may react in a paradoxical fashion becoming irritable and restless.

## PSYCHIC STIMULANTS

Dextroamphetamine (Dexedrine) and methylphenidate (Ritalin) are effective in calming some hyperactive children. The dose recommended is 5–20 mg a day, but may be much higher, and is given in the early part of the day to prevent sleep disturbance. For details see p. 164.

## B. BOOKS RELATING TO CHILD PSYCHIATRY

*Introductory Texts*

BARKER P. (1976). *Basic Child Psychiatry*. 2nd ed. London, Crosby, Lockwood, Staples.

BRITISH MEDICAL JOURNAL. (1972). *Emotional Problems of Childhood and Adolescence*. London, British Medical Journal Publications.

CHESS S. (1969). *An Introduction to Child Psychiatry*. 2nd ed. New York, Grune & Stratton.

NURCOMBE B. (1972). *An Outline of Child Psychiatry*. Sydney. New South Wales University Press Ltd.

STONE F.H. & KOUPERNIK C. (1974). *Child Psychiatry for Students*. Edinburgh, Churchill Livingstone.


*Textbooks and Books for reference*

HOWELLS J.G. (ed.). (1965). *Modern Perspectives in Child Psychiatry*. Edinburgh, Oliver and Boyd.

HOWELLS J.G. (ed.). (1969). *Modern Perspectives in International Child Psychiatry*. Edinburgh, Oliver and Boyd.

HOWELLS J.G. (ed.). (1971). *Modern Perspectives in Adolescent Psychiatry* Edinburgh, Oliver and Boyd.

KANNER L. (1972). *Child Psychiatry*. 4th ed. Springfield, Illinois, Charles C. Thomas.

MILLER E. (1968). *Foundations of Child Psychiatry*. Oxford, Pergamon Press.

RUTTER M. & HERSOV L. (eds) (1977). *Child Psychiatry: Modern Approaches*. Oxford, Blackwell Scientific Publications.

SHAW C.R. & LUCAS A.R. (1970). *The Psychiatric Disorders of Childhood*. 2nd ed. London, Butterworths.

SHIRLEY H.F. (1963). *Paediatric Psychiatry*. Cambridge, Massachusetts, Harvard University Press.

TALBOT N.B., KAGAN J. & EISENBERG L. (1971). *Behavioural Science in Paediatric Medicine*. Philadelphia, London, Toronto, W.B. Saunders Co.

WERRY J.S., QUAY H.C. (eds) (1972). *The Psychopathological Disorders of Childhood*. New York, Wiley.

*Relevant sections in general psychiatric texts:*

FREEDMAN A.M., KAPLAN H.I. & SADOCK B. (1975). 2nd ed. *Comprehensive Textbook of Psychiatry.* Baltimore: Williams and Wilkins Co.
SLATER E. & ROTH M. (1969). Mayer-Gross, Slater & Roth. *Clinical Psychiatry.* 3rd ed. London, Baillière, Tindall and Cassell Ltd.

*Other reading*

BARKER P. (ed.). (1974). *The Residential Psychiatric Treatment of Children.* London, Crosby Lockwood Staples.
BOWLBY J. (1971). *Attachment and Loss.* Vol **1**. *Attachment,* Vol **2**. *Separation – Anxiety & Anger.* Ringwood, Victoria, Penguin Books Australia Ltd.
FREUD A. (1973). *Normality and Pathology in Childhood.* Ringwood, Victoria, Australia. Penguin Books Australia Ltd.
SEGAL H. (1975). *An Introduction to the Work of MelanieKlein.* London, Hogarth Press.
WOLF S. (1973). 2nd ed. *Children under Stress.* Ringwood, Victoria. Penguin Books Australia Ltd.

*\*A very useful source of information relating to new work.*

CHESS S. & THOMAS A. (eds.). (1968–76). *Annual Progress in Child Psychiatry and Child Development.* New York, Brunner Mazel.

This series of books is published yearly and consists of selected republished papers. Where papers cited in the reference lists following each chapter are reprinted in this series, the original source is quoted but this series is also cited thus: *Annual Progress, Vol, Year published.

*Journals*

*The Journal of Child Psychology and Psychiatry* – Pergamon Press for the Association of Child Psychology and Psychiatry. Published 4 times a year.
*The American Journal of Orthopsychiatry* – American Orthopsychiatric Association. Published 4 times a year.
*Developmental Medicine and Child Neurology.* Spastics International Medical Publications. Published 6 times a year.

# Index

Psychotherapy
  in autism  183
  child, benefits  11

Queensland test  64

Rationalisation as defence mechanism
  104
Reaction formation as defence
  mechanism  104, 105
Reactive disorder (adaption reaction)
  44
Reading
  difficulties  171-2
  antisocial behaviour  172
  terminology  171
  tests  66-7
Regression as defence mechanism
  104
Repression as defence mechanism
  104
Risk factors, recognition  16
Ritualistic behaviour as defence
  mechanism  104
Rocking  153
Rorschach Test  68
Rubella, congenital
  and autism  182
  mental subnormality  193

Schizophrenia
  in adolescence  206-7
  in childhood  48, 179
  recognition  3
Schonell Arithmetic Attainment and
  Diagnostic test  67
Schonell Attainment and Diagnostic
  tests of reading  66
Schonell Diagnostic English Tests
  67
School
  absence  109-12, 121-2
  chronic physical illness  109
  and family problems  109
  refusal  110-12
  example  121-2
  in older children  112
  pattern  110
  phobia  110
  treatment  111
  truancy  110
  attendance made compulsory  4

child, disturbed, programmes  18
primary and child's development
  34-5
psychiatric disturbance during
  37-8
problems  10
work, difficulties with  170
Sedatives in childhood  219
Self-stimulating behaviour  153
Sexual
  deviations  113
  role in adolescence  200
Sleep disturbance, older children
  151-2
  pre-school child  150-1
Social
  adjustment in adolescence  201-2
  development  27
  vs emotional deprivation  87-8
  worker involvement  14
Socio-cultural deprivation  86-7
  example  92-3
  prevention  88
Somatic symptoms in neurosis  107
Speech
  disorders  44, 161-2
  pathology  161-2
  therapy  13
Spina bifida  141
Stammering as developmental
  disorder  44
Stanford Binet Intelligence Scale
  63-4
Step-parents  86
Stimulation, genital  153
Stranger anxiety  33
Stress
  children's reaction  100-24
  types of response  100-1
  as precipitating factor in
  psychophysiological disorder
  126
Suicide in adolescence  211-12
Symptom substitution  6
Syphilis and mental subnormality
  193

Teaching, special  4
Television violence  90
Tension discharge disorder  113
  example  122-4
Terminal illness in children,
  management  142-3
  clinical example  146-7